Mental disorders:

Glossary and guide to their classification in accordance with the Ninth Revision of the International Classification of Diseases

World Health Organization   Geneva   1978

Reprinted, 1980, with minor corrections
Second reimpression, 1981

ISBN 92 4 154137 7

PRINTED IN SWITZERLAND

81/5131 – Presses Centrales – 5000

Contents

Participants in the preparation of the volume

Miss E. M. Brooke, formerly Head, Department of Medical Statistics, University Institute of Social and Preventive Medicine, Lausanne, Switzerland (Annex 3).

Dr J. E. Cooper, Professor of Psychiatry, University of Nottingham Medical School, Nottingham, England (section on "The nature of Chapter V..."; quick reference lists; editorial organization).

Dr A. Jablensky, Senior Medical Officer, Division of Mental Health, World Health Organization (overall coordination).

Dr M. Kramer, Professor, Department of Mental Hygiene, Johns Hopkins University, School of Hygiene and Public Health, Baltimore, MD, USA (Annexes 1 and 2).

Dr N. Sartorius, Director, Division of Mental Health, World Health Organization (overall coordination).

Acknowledgements

Simultaneously with work leading to the finalization of the glossary issued for use with ICD-8, the international group of experts which met annually at the seminars held between 1965 and 1972, and listed in the Preface, made proposals which served as the basis for the revision of Chapter V of ICD-9. The draft of the revised Chapter V, with glossary incorporated, was circulated to the members of the WHO Expert Panel on Mental Health and other experts in more than 60 countries, who made valuable comments and suggestions. Those comments and suggestions, systematized and summarized by WHO, in collaboration with Dr M. Rutter, Professor of Child Psychiatry, London, and Dr J. E. Cooper, Professor of Psychiatry, University of Nottingham Medical School, Nottingham, England,were used in the preparation of the final version, adopted by the International Conference for the Ninth Revision of the International Classification of Diseases (Geneva, 1975).

Foreword

This brief foreword was written by the late Sir Aubrey Lewis for the Glossary of Mental Disorders and Guide to their Classification *that was issued in 1974 for use in conjunction with the Eighth Revision of the International Classification of Diseases. It is reproduced here in recognition of Sir Aubrey's fundamental contribution to that glossary, which constitutes the core of the glossary that is now an official part of the mental disorders chapter of the Ninth Revision.*

Compiling glossaries has been a respectable profession since the 2nd century B.C., as the article in the Encyclopaedia Britannica makes abundantly clear. This is not surprising when the multifarious needs for classification and interpretation are considered. But there is a reverse side to the coin: to "gloss over", or "to gloze", a term derived from the same root as glossary, denotes a disreputable activity. "Classification" likewise has a pejorative as well as a respectable flavour. Psychiatric usage of the relevant terms attests their ambiguity: "mere labelling", "the neat complacency of classification", "nosological stamp collecting", "a medical hortus siccus". Such damning phrases arise in part from revulsion against the excesses to which classification was pushed in the late 18th and early 19th century.

A modern psychiatric glossarist has to cope basically with the same uncertainties and pitfalls as beset the compilers of other medical classifications, but they are aggravated by hazards arising from the paucity of the objective data on which definition and diagnosis must depend. He has to contrive appropriate criteria for differentiating one disease from another; ideally he aims at constructing a consistent schema into which they will all fit. Such a schema may be based on clinical patterns (syndromes) or on clinical course; it may be psychodynamic, etiological (genetic), or pathological. And, since diseases are in any case abstract concepts, it is no wonder that the disease constructs which psychiatrists work with have shimmering outlines and overlap. Observer variation is disconcertingly in evidence; reliability is too low for scientific comfort; discrepancies may be in some cases lessened, in others minimized, depending on whether they arise from inexact perception, personal bias, or divergency of the nosological systems or terms used.

The picture is no longer black. The glossary put forward here, when faithfully applied, reduces the scope of error. It would seem, however, that accurate observation is still the gate that needs the closest guard. A. R. Feinstein put it bluntly: "the current psychiatric debates about systems of classification, the many hypothetical and unconfirmed schemas of " psychodynamic mechanisms", and the concern with etiological inference rather than observational evidence are nosologic activities sometimes reminiscent of those conducted by the mediaeval taxonomists." Since the disorders listed in this glossary are identified by criteria that are predominantly descriptive, its use should encourage an emphasis on careful observation.

This glossary still contains some compromises and anomalies, but the emergence of an agreed version from an international group of collaborators and advisers of such diversity of background and outlook was possible only because of a generous spirit of cooperation and common recognition of an urgent need for better means of communication.

Sir Aubrey J. Lewis, M.D., F.R.C.P.
1974

Preface

This volume is a successor to the Glossary of Mental Disorders and Guide to their Classification *that was issued for use in conjunction with Chapter V (Mental Disorders) of the Eighth Revision of the International Classification of Diseases (ICD-8),*[1] *and like it, is published for the guidance and convenience both of clinical diagnosticians and of others who may be concerned with the coding of psychiatric information.*

The Ninth Revision of the International Classification of Diseases (ICD-9)[2] *did not bring about fundamental changes in the classification categories in Chapter V, and those already familiar with the Eighth Revision will find the Ninth reasonably similar in outline, although containing a variety of improvements. A major new feature, however, is the inclusion of the glossary of mental disorders as an integral part of Chapter V of ICD-9, in recognition of the relative lack of independent information upon which psychiatric diagnoses are based and the consequent differences in the usage of psychiatric terms in different countries.*

The introductory sections of the previous volume have been brought up to date for the present publication. They are presented in somewhat modified form in the section on the nature and use of Chapter V of ICD-9, which also includes a discussion of the principal differences between ICD-8 and ICD-9.

The next section reproduces in its entirety Chapter V (Mental Disorders) of ICD-9 with the now integrated glossary. This is followed by three Quick Reference Lists designed to minimize the problems of becoming familiar with the novel features of ICD-9. Quick Reference List No. 1, on depressive disorders, should be particularly useful, since there are now 10 3-digit and 19 4-digit categories by means of which various types of depression can be coded. This increase does more justice to the ubiquitous nature of depressive symptoms, but the user still needs a guide when approaching Chapter V initially.

Annexes 1 and 2 give an introduction to and an outline of the whole of ICD-9. Annex 3 lists the 3- and 4-digit categories for those conditions in ICD-9 but outside Chapter V that are most likely to be needed by those

---

[1] WORLD HEALTH ORGANIZATION. *Glossary of mental disorders and guide to their classification, for use in conjunction with the International Classification of Diseases, 8th revision,* Geneva, 1974.

[2] WORLD HEALTH ORGANIZATION. *Manual of the International Statistical Classification of Diseases, Injuries, and Causes of Death,* 1975 (Ninth) Revision, Geneva, Volumes 1 and 2, 1977 and 1978.

who collect and code psychiatric information. Annex 3 should allow the user to cope with the great majority of instances where two codes are required, and only occasional reference to the full ICD-9 volumes will be needed.

Finally, an alphabetical index of the headings of categories, of sub-categories and of other recommended terms in Chapter V of ICD-9 and in Annex 3 is provided for quick reference.

Changes and new categories in the International Classification of Diseases have been introduced only for sound reasons and after much consideration. As far as possible, the changes in Chapter V have been based upon evidence that the new codes function better than the old ones. Some of this evidence, and a large proportion of the other changes based upon discussion and consideration of different viewpoints, emanated from the World Health Organization's programme on the standardization of psychiatric diagnosis, classification and statistics. A central feature of this programme was a series of eight international seminars held annually between 1965 and 1972, each of which focussed upon a recognized problem area in psychiatric diagnosis. Psychiatrists from more than 40 countries participated, and the documents and proposals that were used to produce the recommendations for ICD-9 in the eighth and final seminar were seen and commented upon by many more.

The following seminars were held, the first seven focussing on the classification of major groups of psychiatric disorders, and the last seminar on programme review: [1]

Place	Year	Subject
London	1965	Functional psychoses, with emphasis on schizophrenia
Oslo	1966	Borderline psychosis, reactive psychosis
Paris	1967	Psychiatric disorders of childhood
Moscow	1968	Mental disorders of old age
Washington, D C	1969	Mental retardation
Basle	1970	Neurotic and psychosomatic disorders
Tokyo	1971	Personality disorder and drug addiction
Geneva	1972	Summary, conclusions, recommendations and proposals for further research

This volume is thus the product of an international collaborative effort and the fruit of much debate and constructive discussion. It is hoped that its users will find it helpful and will continue to assist WHO in the further development of the glossary by providing their comments and suggestions.

---

[1] A list of published material and reports on these seminars is available from the World Health Organization, upon request.

The nature of Chapter V (Mental Disorders) of the ICD-9, and how to use it

Nomenclatures, classifications and glossaries

To obtain the maximum benefit from using the Ninth Revision of the International Classification of Diseases (ICD-9), and the glossary incorporated in its Chapter V, and to apply it with the greatest possible consistency, it is necessary to understand some basic points about systems of classification of diseases. The classification of diseases cannot begin without a list of agreed names of diseases in which each name stands for only one disease; such a list is called a *nomenclature*. Since a nomenclature is merely a list carrying no implications about the relationships between its constituent terms, agreed names of new illnesses can simply be added as they are identified without affecting the terms already present.

The next step is to group together these names according to stated criteria so that diseases with properties in common are brought together in classes; such a grouping is called a *classification*. The nature of the criteria upon which the classes are formed will depend upon the purposes of the classification—there is no one single type of classification that suits all purposes. In general medicine a classification by cause is very useful for many purposes, but in psychiatry the causes of the majority of mental illnesses are still poorly understood. Consequently, other criteria have to be relied upon, such as similarity of symptoms and behaviour, or course of illness. When a new illness is added to an already established classification, care must be taken to ensure that it is placed in correct relationship to other similar conditions, depending upon the criteria being used in that particular classification. (This is in contrast to a nomenclature, to which one can simply add new illnesses without having to consider such relationships). An additional complication in classifications designed primarily for statistical purposes, such as the ICD, is that each section is initially allotted a fixed number of categories. When a statistical classification is first set up, all the terms in the existing nomenclature have to be fitted into these categories. Since it is often impossible to leave spaces for future changes or additions, the insertion of a new term may require the elimination of other terms or the rearrangement of already accepted parts of the classification. It is therefore often necessary to adopt a comparatively conservative attitude to suggestions for changes in a statistical classification.

No classification of diseases can be used satisfactorily unless some indication is given of the meaning of its constituent terms. A set of descriptions, and if possible definitions, of the terms making up a classification is a *glossary*. Again, there are special problems in psychiatry.

The glossary in the mental health chapter of the ICD-9, reproduced in this book, is necessarily composed of descriptions of symptom patterns and syndromes rather than clear-cut or mutually exclusive definitions. This is because diagnosis by means of a few pathognomonic signs or symptoms is uncommon in psychiatry; in most instances, psychiatric disorders are differentiated from one another by the recognition of different patterns of emphasis among a comparatively small number of symptoms.

The ICD

The various revisions of the ICD have always had as their primary aim the classification of morbidity and mortality information on a national and international scale. The ICD is thus a classification of *diseases,* rather than *patients.* Since one patient may have more than one disease, there must be rules of procedure indicating how the several conditions should be recorded; these rules will vary with the purposes for which the data are being collected. (Several possible sets of rules that might be used in connexion with the mental health glossary in Chapter V of the ICD-9 are summarized on pages 11 to 15).

Although the axes of classification in the ICD-9 vary from one section to the next (see Annex 1, page 62), the psychiatric section is itself a compromise in that the criteria upon which it is based are not uniform throughout, owing to the special problems of psychiatry. Chapter V follows predominantly descriptive lines, but etiological and prognostic criteria are also used in some categories. While this complicates its use, some difficulties of this type are inevitable given the present state of psychiatric knowledge and the need to make the ICD acceptable to as many different countries and schools of thought as possible.

Glossary for use with the psychiatric section of the ICD-9

All the previous revisions of the ICD have been published without any indication of the meanings of the constituent terms. Guidance to Chapter V of the ICD-9 has now been added in the form of a glossary because it has become increasingly obvious that many key psychiatric terms are acquiring very different meanings in different countries. Unless some attempt is made to encourage uniformity of usage of descriptive and diagnostic terms, very little meaning can be attributed to the diagnostic side of statistics of mental illness based upon the ICD, and in many other ways communication between psychiatrists will become increasingly difficult. The glossary necessarily reflects any inconsistencies or difficulties inherent in the arrangement of Chapter V, which, as already noted, must represent a compromise. (The International Conference for the Ninth Revision, held in 1975, noted that standardization of nomenclature on a multilingual basis was essential for conformity in diagnosis and suggested that glossaries similar to that developed for Chapter V might be provided for other specialties where diagnostic concepts were unclear.)

Thus, the main aim of the ICD-9 and glossary is to ensure as far as possible that those who apply it will arrive at a uniform use of the principal diagnostic terms current in psychiatry. In addition to helping to minimize discrepancies among the diagnostic concepts used by psychiatrists in different countries for the statistical reporting of mental illness, use of the ICD-9 and glossary in publications dealing with either clinical issues or research will also assist psychiatrists from different countries and schools of thought in understanding each other's work and concepts.

Apart from its primary purpose of fostering communication, Chapter V of ICD-9 with its glossary can also serve as an educational stimulus, since it was compiled by psychiatrists representing many different countries and points of view. It is unlikely that any one psychiatrist will find that all the terms and descriptions coincide with his own personal views or usage. Disagreements naturally arise from the existence of different viewpoints, each of which has some support. For purposes of communication, however, it is necessary to arrive at a working compromise, and this is what the ICD-9 and glossary represent. They undoubtedly contain some inconsistencies, but the presence of these and the retention of vague terms such as "neurosis" and "psychosis" are rooted in psychiatric custom and history. It is hoped that discussion of these difficult and controversial points will serve to highlight the problems underlying all systems of medical and psychiatric classification, and will emphasize the need to acknowledge and try to understand the opinions of others.

Some specific issues involved in the use of Chapter V of the ICD-9

The glossary in Chapter V has been prepared to give guidance to psychiatrists in selecting the diagnostic code that most nearly describes the clinical characteristics of the patient. It is also designed to be used by coders responsible for assigning diagnoses to the proper ICD-9 categories.

As far as the terms in the ICD-9 permit, the glossary consists merely of descriptions of symptoms or syndromes. Etiological statements and assumptions have been avoided except where a widespread demand for their inclusion became apparent. The major exceptions to this avoidance of etiological statements are (*a*) in categories 290–294, where an organic etiology is implicit in the ICD headings, (*b*) in category 298, "nonorganic" or "psychogenic" psychoses, and (*c*) in the new categories 308 and 309 —"Acute reaction to stress" and "Adjustment reaction", respectively.

When using the ICD and glossary for statistical purposes, the user should avoid making a firm diagnosis in his own terms and then merely searching for the nearest equivalent among the ICD headings. He should familiarize himself with the glossary descriptions in advance and then choose the description that most nearly fits the patient's illness, even if this means selecting a term not personally familiar to the diagnostician or his national colleagues.

It is inevitable that many psychiatrists will find that some of the descriptions and rules of the glossary are in conflict with their own diagnostic preferences. Where they cannot reconcile the glossary descriptions and rules with their own convictions and practice, it is open to them when, for example, reporting their own special research or clinical interests, to modify, enlarge, or regroup the ICD terms—and modify this glossary accordingly—provided that they make it clear how their terms can be converted into those of the glossary and the ICD. In some cases a national glossary can be used with the same proviso, so as to encourage consistency within a given country.

Users of the ICD are urged always to use the exact terms specified as the heading of each category, whether 3-digit or 4-digit. In many cases, other terms are also listed below the glossary description. This implies that the term is recognized as an acceptable and frequently used name for a disease or condition falling into that category, or as an acceptable synonym for the category heading. All 3- and 4-digit headings and inclusion terms appearing in the glossary have been assembled in an alphabetical index (page 83) for quick reference and assistance in assigning diagnoses to the appropriate code. (The Alphabetical Index in Volume 2 of the ICD-9 should be consulted for guidance on how to code terms not found in the present index). Terms considered obsolete or confusing have been purposely excluded from the glossary, however interesting or important their history.

Before the ICD can be used satisfactorily for classifying patients, some provision has to be made for those patients who have more than one diagnosis. The rules of procedure adopted will depend upon the purposes for which the patients are being classified; no single system can be suitable for all purposes. Some examples are given below of commonly used systems of different degrees of complexity. Diagnosticians and other users of the ICD-9 and glossary should always be aware of the requirements and purposes of the recording system to which they are contributing a diagnosis.

Where only one diagnosis can be recorded for each patient, it is often stipulated that the diagnosis most relevant to the reason for admission or contact should be the one recorded. If the reason for admission or contact is not the main interest, then it may be preferable to give one type of diagnosis precedence over others according to a set of hierarchical rules. These rules may be applied by the psychiatrist or by those responsible for analysing the diagnoses. For instance, all organically based psychiatric illnesses may be given precedence over functional ones, and within the functional group the order then may be psychoses, neuroses, personality disorders, and others. Whichever procedure is chosen to fit the particular purpose for which diagnoses are recorded, the rules applied should be made explicit and followed consistently.

Modern data recording systems can usually handle more than one diagnostic statement about each patient, and more than one should be recorded whenever appropriate. Depending upon the reason for collecting the diagnoses, a set of rules of precedence is needed to determine the order in which the diagnoses should be recorded. The hierarchy suggested in the preceding paragraph is often found to be satisfactory for psychiatric purposes. In addition, underlying or associated physical conditions should be recorded by means of separate ICD codes. Those conditions most commonly found in association with psychiatric conditions are listed for convenience in Annex 3, pages 69–82. A list of categories for ill-defined conditions and nonspecific symptoms is also provided (categories 780–799).

The following examples illustrate codings of some double-entry diagnoses.

Diagnosis	Code from ICD-9	Associated condition
Organic psychosis (dementia) in general paralysis of the insane	294.1	094.1
Organic psychosis with arteriosclerosis (arteriosclerotic dementia)	290.4	437.0
Organic psychosis (dementia) with multiple sclerosis	294.1	340
Organic psychosis (dementia) with epilepsy (convulsive)	294.1	345.1
Nonpsychotic mental disorders (e.g., personality changes with convulsive epilepsy)	310.1	345.1
Psychogenic duodenal ulcer	316	532
Mental retardation, moderate, associated with rubella, congenital	318.0	771.0
Mental retardation, severe, associated with lead poisoning	318.1	984
Suicide attempt, barbiturate poisoning, as a result of neurotic depression	300.4	E950.1

Users of the ICD are encouraged to consider using the supplementary E and V codes whenever they apply, so as to increase the recognition of the importance of other nonmedical factors. The E codes are largely unchanged for ICD-9, and the former Y codes, covering factors which influence health status or health service contact but which are not in themselves medical conditions, have been replaced by an extensive set of new V codes. Summary versions of these are presented in Annex 3, but the full text of ICD-9 needs to be consulted for their proper use in detail.

Categories 290–294 ("Organic psychotic conditions") should only be used, as in ICD-8, when the specifically organic clinical features of dementia, delirium or confusional state are present. They should not be used simply to imply the organic etiology of a psychotic mental state that is coded elsewhere in Chapter V. For instance, a postpartum psychosis presenting with the clinical picture of schizophrenia and exhibiting none of the specified organic features ("impairment of orientation, memory, comprehension, calculation, learning capacity and judgement") should be classified under 295, "Schizophrenic psychoses", and a separate entry made for the associated physical condition of childbirth (V27).

If a recording system is required that allows some indication of diagnostic certainties and uncertainties, then a great deal of information can be contained in a triple system in which Main, Subsidiary, and Alternative Diagnoses are recorded. In such a system, the Main Diagnosis is the one most relevant to the purpose of collection of the statistics. This may be all that is necessary, particularly in clear-cut and severe mental illnesses. If another psychiatric condition is present in addition to the main diagnosis, a Subsidiary Diagnosis is recorded; this does not conflict with the Main Diagnosis but describes additional features (for example, Main Diagnosis: Schizophrenia, schizo-affective type; Subsidiary Diagnosis: Personality disorder, anankastic). If there is any serious uncertainty about the Main Diagnosis, an Alternative Diagnosis is also recorded (e.g., Main Diagnosis: Manic-depressive psychosis, manic type; Subsidiary Diagnosis: none; Alternative Diagnosis: Schizophrenia, schizo-affective type). This or similar methods can be used to identify those diagnoses that are particularly liable to lead to disagreements among psychiatrists. Further studies can then be designed to show whether the disagreements originated from poor definition of the psychiatric condition or from different interpretations or usages of the definition.

Many other systems are possible, and these examples are given merely to encourage users of the ICD and glossary to make sure that they understand the purposes for which their diagnoses are being made.

These notes should make it clear that the aim of the glossary is not to impose theoretical concepts upon the user in his clinical or research work but simply to guide him in classifying mental disorders for purposes of international coding and communication with others. Once this fundamental point has been accepted, doctors will realize how important it is to use the exact ICD term when recording their diagnosis on forms or documents to be used later by clerical and administrative staff who have not had medical training. Even a slight variation from the ICD heading may be confusing for coders who cannot be expected to know how to interpret the personal diagnostic terms or systems of individual doctors.

An outline of the differences in the mental health chapter between the Eighth (1965) Revision and the Ninth (1975) Revision of the International Classification of Diseases is given on pages 19–20, where the 3-digit categories for ICD-8 and ICD-9 are set side by side. It will be seen from that list that ICD-9 is not radically different from ICD-8, but that there are certain changes that call for explanatory comment.

Differences between Chapter V of ICD-8 and ICD-9

The main changes concern:
(*a*) Depression
(*b*) Disorders of childhood and adolescence
(*c*) Adjustment and stress reactions
(*d*) Psychic factors associated with diseases classified elsewhere
(*e*) Organic psychotic conditions
(*f*) Other categories.

(*a*) *Depression.* The dichotomy between neurotic and psychotic disorders, which has always caused problems in the classification of depressive disorders, could not be abandoned in ICD-9. However, the position has been improved by an increase in the number of categories which refer to different varieties of depression. The increase (from 10 to 19 categories at a 4-digit level) comes from a more sensible arrangement of affective psychoses, from the new approach to transient disorders, and from the proper provision of categories for disorders of childhood and adolescence. In view of the frequency with which depressive disorders need to be coded, all 3- and 4-digit categories covering some aspect of depression have been grouped together in Quick Reference List No. 1, on page 58.

Category 311, "Depressive disorder, not elsewhere classified" is provided to try to cope with an unfortunately common problem that often faces those attempting to code the too general diagnostic statements of others. A simple statement of "depression" and "depressive illness" is still all too frequently to be found on case notes as the sole diagnostic indication; such disorders should be coded to this category, thereby preserving as much as possible the meaning of other categories for depressive illnesses clearly specified as neurotic or psychotic. Category 311 also provides a solution for those clinicians who believe that depressive illnesses occur which cannot be satisfactorily classified in ICD terms as either neurotic or psychotic.

(b) *Disorders of childhood and adolescence.* A lack of specific provision for these was a major defect of ICD-8. Four major 3-digit categories (and their 22 4-digit subdivisions) are now provided in ICD-9 (see Quick Reference List No. 2). These are: 299, "Psychoses with origin specific to childhood" (principally infantile autism and disintegrative psychosis); 313, "Disturbance of emotions specific to childhood and adolescence" (subdivided according to the predominant type of emotion); 314, "Hyperkinetic syndrome of childhood"; and 315, "Specific delays in development". Some of the subdivisions of other new 3-digit categories are also often applicable to children; for instance, some varieties of 309, "Adjustment reaction", and of 312, "Disturbance of conduct not elsewhere classified". Enuresis, encopresis and stammering are subdivisions of 307, "Special symptoms or syndromes not elsewhere classified".

(c) *Adjustment and stress reactions.* ICD-8 contained category 307, "Transient situational disturbances", but this was not well defined and was not subdivided. Psychiatrists are required to deal more and more with individuals who do not fit the criteria for neurotic or psychotic illnesses, but who are in abnormal (although transient) states of emotional disturbance. Two new 3-digit categories have now been provided, each with several subdivisions. Category 308, "Acute reaction to stress", applies to transient states apparently induced by unusually severe mental or physical stress. Category 309, "Adjustment reaction", is intended for use when the reaction is more prolonged, usually in response to stress of a less spectacular nature and a longer duration.

(d) *Psychic factors associated with diseases classified elsewhere.* The term " psychosomatic " was considered unsatisfactory for this category, although often used in this connexion.

Category 316 provides a new and simple method of recording an association between psychological processes or events or stress and an identifiable physical condition that has a code elsewhere. Use of 316 simply implies the presence of such an association without more detailed specification, and a second code is then used to identify the specific physical condition. For instance, a patient with asthma regarded as psychogenic would be coded to 316 and 493.9. It should be noted, however, that autonomic nervous system symptoms not involving tissue damage and some other less well defined symptoms and syndromes do not qualify for the use of 316, and should be coded to 306 and 307 respectively. With respect to asthma, for instance, this new system avoids a problem created by category 305 in ICD-8 in which such "psychosomatic" conditions could be coded either under Chapter V or under the chapter for respiratory diseases.

(*e*) *Organic psychotic conditions.* The classification of these has been simplified, largely by leaving out the categories 292, 293 and 294 of ICD-8 in which a large number of specific physical conditions were listed as causing organic psychotic states. In ICD-9 a separate code from another chapter should be used if a cause is known for an organic psychotic condition. The organic psychotic condition itself can now be further specified as dementia of various types (290), as transient (293), or as other more chronic varieties (294).

(*f*) *Other categories.* The only other new 3-digit category not already mentioned is 305, "Nondependent abuse of drugs". The number of 3-digit categories reserved for mental retardation has been reduced from 6 to 3, but this will not result in any lack of etiological information if the principle is followed of using additional separate codes from elsewhere in the ICD to specify associated physical conditions.

Dual classification (dagger and asterisk codes)

This is a new feature of ICD-9 which does not occur in Chapter V, but an explanatory note is needed since users will encounter these symbols in other chapters of the classification, particularly in Chapter VI ("Diseases of the Nervous System and Sense Organs"). Some diagnoses which contain two pieces of information have been provided with two separate code numbers in different positions in the classification. Usually one of these is to do with an underlying disease process; following the normal ICD practice, this is regarded as the primary position. The dagger symbol (†) indicates this. The secondary position is in that part of the classification dealing with the organ system to which the manifestation or complication is related, and is marked with an asterisk (*). For example, tuberculous meningitis has its primary code number in Chapter I ("Infectious and parasitic diseases"), marked with a dagger (013.0†) and another in Chapter VI ("Diseases of the nervous system and sense organs") marked with an asterisk (320.4*). The primary or dagger position of these dual codes is always the one to be recorded when additional codes are needed to supplement a code from Chapter V.

ICD-9 and other classifications and glossaries

The existence of the ICD-9 as a means of international communication does not prevent the development of separate national classifications and glossaries. It is to be hoped, however, that the compilers of separate systems will always ensure compatibility or equivalence between their systems and the ICD, to everyone's advantage.

The World Health Organization would appreciate receiving comments and suggestions from users of the ICD-9, particularly from those who are able to test out the categories in systematic investigations.[1] Comments on both general and specific points will be considered when revising the classification and glossary. Preliminary work on collecting suggestions and information for the Tenth Revision of the ICD is already starting, and it is hoped that its final form will be the result of much international discussion and collaboration.

---

[1] Comments and suggestions concerning mental disorders should be addressed to: Division of Mental Health, World Health Organization, 1211 Geneva 27, Switzerland.

Offprint of Chapter V (Mental Disorders) of the ICD-9

Chapter V (Mental Disorders) of the ICD-9 is offprinted on the following pages (pages 21 to 57).

The 3-digit categories of Chapter V are listed in the right-hand column below so that the reader can see at a glance how this chapter is arranged; the page numbers shown lead to the 4-digit subcategories and to the descriptions of terms that constitute the glossary.

For the convenience of those who have been accustomed to using the ICD-8, the left-hand column shows how the ICD-8 categories compare with those in the new ICD-9.

Mental Disorders as Classified in the ICD-8

MENTAL RETARDATION (310–315)

310 Borderline mental retardation
311 Mild mental retardation
312 Moderate mental retardation
313 Severe mental retardation
314 Profound mental retardation
315 Unspecified mental retardation

Mental Disorders as Classified in the IC[

NEUROTIC DISORDERS *(continued)*

310 Specific nonpsychotic mental disorders following organic brain damage . . . .
311 Depressive disorder, not elsewhere classified . . . .
312 Disturbance of conduct not elsewhere classified . . . .
313 Disturbance of emotions specific to childhood and adolescence . . . .
314 Hyperkinetic syndrome of childhood . .
315 Specific delays in development . . . .
316 Psychic factors associated with diseases classified elsewhere . . . .

MENTAL RETARDATION (317–319)

317 Mild mental retardation . . . .
318 Other specified mental retardation . .
319 Unspecified mental retardation . . . .

V. MENTAL DISORDERS

This section of the Classification differs from the others in that it includes a glossary, prepared after consultation with experts from many different countries, defining the contents of the rubrics.   This difference is considered to be justified because of the special problems posed for psychiatrists by the relative lack of independent laboratory information upon which to base their diagnoses.   The diagnosis of many of the most important mental disorders still relies largely upon descriptions of abnormal experience and behaviour, and without some guidance in the form of a glossary that can serve as a common frame of reference, psychiatric communications easily become unsatisfactory at both clinical and statistical levels.

Many well-known terms have different meanings in current use, and it is important for the user to use the glossary descriptions and not merely the category titles when searching for the best fit for the condition he is trying to code.   This is particularly important if a separate national glossary also exists.

The instructions "Use additional code to identify..." are important because of the nature of many psychiatric conditions in which two or more codes are necessary to describe the condition and the associated or causal factors.   It should be used whenever possible.

In cases where no other information is available except that a mental disorder is present, the code V40.9 (unspecified mental or behavioural problems) can be used.

Psychoses (290-299)

Mental disorders in which impairment of mental function has developed to a degree that interferes grossly with insight, ability to meet some ordinary demands of life or to maintain adequate contact with reality.   It is not an exact or well defined term. Mental retardation is excluded.

Organic psychotic conditions (290-294)

Syndromes in which there is impairment of orientation, memory, comprehension, calculation, learning capacity and judgement.   These are the essential features but there may also be shallowness or lability of affect, or a more persistent disturbance of mood, lowering of ethical standards and exaggeration or emergence of personality traits, and diminished capacity for independent decision.

Psychoses of the types classifiable to 295-298 and without the above features are excluded even though they may be associated with organic conditions.

The term '*dementia*' in this glossary includes organic psychoses as just specified, of a chronic or progressive nature, which if untreated are usually irreversible and terminal.

The term '*delirium*' in this glossary includes organic psychoses with a short course in which the above features are overshadowed by clouded consciousness, confusion, disorientation, delusions, illusions and often vivid hallucinations.

Includes: psychotic organic brain syndrome

Excludes: nonpsychotic syndromes of organic aetiology (see 310.–)
            psychoses classifiable to 295-298 and without the above
            features but associated with physical disease, injury, or
            condition affecting the brain [e.g., following childbirth];
            code to 295-298 and use additional code to identify the
            associated physical condition

290   Senile and presenile organic psychotic conditions

Excludes: psychoses classifiable to 295-298.8 occurring in the senium
            without dementia or delirium (295-298)
            transient organic psychotic conditions (293.–)
            dementia not classified as senile, presenile, or arteriosclerotic
            (294.1)

290.0   *Senile dementia, simple type*

Dementia occurring usually after the age of 65 in which any cerebral pathology other
than that of senile atrophic change can be reasonably excluded.

Excludes: mild memory disturbances, not amounting to dementia,
            associated with senile brain disease (310.1)
            senile dementia:
                depressed or paranoid type (290.2)
                with confusion and/or delirium (290.3)

290.1   *Presenile dementia*

Dementia occurring usually before the age of 65 in patients with the relatively rare
forms of diffuse or lobar cerebral atrophy. Use additional code to identify the associated neurological condition.

Brain syndrome with presenile brain disease
Circumscribed atrophy of the brain
Dementia in:
  Alzheimer's disease
  Pick's disease of the brain

Excludes: arteriosclerotic dementia (290.4)
            dementia associated with other cerebral conditions (294.1)

290.2   *Senile dementia, depressed or paranoid type*

A type of senile dementia characterized by development in advanced old age, progressive
in nature, in which a variety of delusions and hallucinations of a persecutory, depressive
and somatic content are also present. Disturbance of the sleep/waking cycle and
preoccupation with dead people are often particularly prominent.

Senile psychosis NOS

Excludes: senile dementia:
                NOS (290.0)
                with confusion and/or delirium (290.3)

290.3   *Senile dementia with acute confusional state*

Senile dementia with a superimposed reversible episode of acute confusional state

Excludes: senile:
        dementia NOS (290.0)
        psychosis NOS (290.2)

290.4   *Arteriosclerotic dementia*

Dementia attributable, because of physical signs [on examination of the central nervous
system] to degenerative arterial disease of the brain. Symptoms suggesting a focal
lesion in the brain are common. There may be a fluctuating or patchy intellectual
defect with insight, and an intermittent course is common. Clinical differentiation
from senile or presenile dementia, which may coexist with it, may be very difficult or
impossible. Use additional code to identify cerebral atherosclerosis (437.0).

Excludes: suspected cases with no clear evidence of arteriosclerosis
        (290.9)

290.8   *Other*

290.9   *Unspecified*

291   Alcoholic psychoses

Organic psychotic states due mainly to excessive consumption of alcohol; defects of
nutrition are thought to play an important role. In some of these states, withdrawal
of alcohol can be of aetiological significance.

Excludes: alcoholism without psychosis (303)

291.0   *Delirium tremens*

Acute or subacute organic psychotic states in alcoholics, characterized by clouded
consciousness, disorientation, fear, illusions, delusions, hallucinations of any kind,
notably visual and tactile, and restlessness, tremor and sometimes fever.

Alcoholic delirium

291.1   *Korsakov's psychosis, alcoholic*

A syndrome of prominent and lasting reduction of memory span, including striking
loss of recent memory, disordered time appreciation and confabulation, occurring in
alcoholics as the sequel to an acute alcoholic psychosis [especially delirium tremens]
or, more rarely, in the course of chronic alcoholism. It is usually accompanied by
peripheral neuritis and may be associated with Wernicke's encephalopathy.

Alcoholic polyneuritic psychosis

Excludes: Korsakov's psychosis:
        NOS (294.0)
        nonalcoholic (294.0)

291.2   *Other alcoholic dementia*

Nonhallucinatory dementias occurring in association with alcoholism but not characterized by the features of either delirium tremens or Korsakov's psychosis.

Alcoholic dementia NOS
Chronic alcoholic brain syndrome

291.3   *Other alcoholic hallucinosis*

A psychosis usually of less than six months' duration, with slight or no clouding of consciousness and much anxious restlessness in which auditory hallucinations, mostly of voices uttering insults and threats, predominate.

Excludes: schizophrenia (295.–) and paranoid states (297.–) taking the
            form of chronic hallucinosis with clear consciousness in
            an alcoholic

291.4   *Pathological drunkenness*

Acute psychotic episodes induced by relatively small amounts of alcohol. These are regarded as individual idiosyncratic reactions to alcohol, not due to excessive consumption and without conspicuous neurological signs of intoxication.

Excludes: simple drunkenness (305.0)

291.5   *Alcoholic jealousy*

Chronic paranoid psychosis characterized by delusional jealousy and associated with alcoholism.

Alcoholic paranoia

Excludes: nonalcoholic paranoid states (297.–)
            schizophrenia, paranoid type (295.3)

291.8   *Other*

Alcohol withdrawal syndrome

Excludes: delirium tremens (291.0)

291.9   *Unspecified*

Alcoholic:
  mania NOS
  psychosis NOS
Alcoholism (chronic) with psychosis

292   **Drug psychoses**

Syndromes that do not fit the descriptions given in 295-298 (nonorganic psychoses) and which are due to consumption of drugs [notably amphetamines, barbiturates and the opiate and LSD groups] and solvents. Some of the syndromes in this group are not as severe as most conditions labelled "psychotic" but they are included here for practical reasons. Use additional E Code to identify the drug and also code drug dependence (304.—) if present.

292.0 *Drug withdrawal syndrome*

States associated with drug withdrawal ranging from severe, as specified for alcohol under 291.0 (delirium tremens) to less severe states characterized by one or more symptoms such as convulsions, tremor, anxiety, restlessness, gastrointestinal and muscular complaints, and mild disorientation and memory disturbance.

292.1 *Paranoid and/or hallucinatory states induced by drugs*

States of more than a few days but not usually of more than a few months duration, associated with large or prolonged intake of drugs, notably of the amphetamine and LSD groups. Auditory hallucinations usually predominate, and there may be anxiety and restlessness.

Excludes: the described conditions with confusion or delirium (293.–)
states following LSD or other hallucinogens, lasting only a few days or less ["bad trips"] (305.3)

292.2 *Pathological drug intoxication*

Individual idiosyncratic reactions to comparatively small quantities of a drug, which take the form of acute, brief psychotic states of any type.

Excludes: physiological side-effects of drugs [e.g., dystonias]
expected brief psychotic reactions to hallucinogens ["bad trips"] (305.3)

292.8 *Other*

292.9 *Unspecified*

293 Transient organic psychotic conditions

States characterized by clouded consciousness, confusion, disorientation, illusions and often vivid hallucinations. They are usually due to some intra- or extracerebral toxic, infectious, metabolic or other systemic disturbance and are generally reversible. Depressive and paranoid symptoms may also be present but are not the main feature. Use additional code to identify the associated physical or neurological condition.

Excludes: confusional state or delirium superimposed on senile dementia (290.3)
dementia due to:
alcohol (291.–)
arteriosclerosis (290.4)
senility (290.0)

293.0 *Acute confusional state*

Short-lived states, lasting hours or days, of the above type.

Acute:
  delirium
  infective psychosis
  organic reaction
  post-traumatic organic
      psychosis

Acute:
  psycho-organic syndrome
  psychosis associated with endo-
      crine, metabolic or cerebro-
      vascular disorder
Epileptic:
  confusional state
  twilight state

293.1   Subacute confusional state

States of the above type in which the symptoms, usually less florid, last for several weeks or longer, during which they may show marked fluctuations in intensity.

Subacute:
  delirium
  infective psychosis
  organic reaction
  post-traumatic organic psychosis

Subacute:
  psycho-organic syndrome
  psychosis associated with endo-
    crine or metabolic disorder

293.8   Other

293.9   Unspecified

294   Other organic psychotic conditions (chronic)

294.0   Korsakov's psychosis or syndrome (nonalcoholic)

Syndromes as described under 291.1 but not due to alcohol.

294.1   Dementia in conditions classified elsewhere

Dementia not classifiable as senile, presenile or arteriosclerotic (290.–) but associated with other underlying conditions.

Dementia in:
  cerebral lipidoses
  epilepsy
  general paralysis of the insane
  hepatolenticular degeneration
  Huntington's chorea
  multiple sclerosis
  polyarteritis nodosa

Use additional code to identify the underlying physical condition

294.8   Other

States that fulfill the criteria of an organic psychosis but do not take the form of a confusional state (293.–), a nonalcoholic Korsakov's psychosis (294.0) or a dementia (294.1).

Mixed paranoid and affective
  organic psychotic states

Epileptic psychosis NOS (code
  also 345.–)

Excludes: mild memory disturbances, not amounting to dementia
             (310.1)

294.9   Unspecified

OTHER PSYCHOSES (295-299)

295   Schizophrenic psychoses

A group of psychoses in which there is a fundamental disturbance of personality, a characteristic distortion of thinking, often a sense of being controlled by alien forces, delusions which may be bizarre, disturbed perception, abnormal affect out of keeping with the real situation, and autism. Nevertheless, clear consciousness and intellectual capacity are usually maintained. The disturbance of personality involves its most basic functions which give the normal person his feeling of individuality, uniqueness and self-direction. The most intimate thoughts, feelings and acts are often felt to be known to or shared by others and explanatory delusions may develop, to the effect that natural or supernatural forces are at work to influence the schizophrenic person's thoughts and actions in ways that are often bizarre. He may see himself as the pivot of all that happens. Hallucinations, especially of hearing, are common and may comment on the patient or address him. Perception is frequently disturbed in other ways; there may be perplexity, irrelevant features may become all-important and, accompanied by passivity feelings, may lead the patient to believe that everyday objects and situations possess a special, usually sinister, meaning intended for him. In the characteristic schizophrenic disturbance of thinking, peripheral and irrelevant features of a total concept, which are inhibited in normal directed mental activity, are brought to the forefront and utilized in place of the elements relevant and appropriate to the situation. Thus thinking becomes vague, elliptical and obscure, and its expression in speech sometimes incomprehensible. Breaks and interpolations in the flow of consecutive thought are frequent, and the patient may be convinced that his thoughts are being withdrawn by some outside agency. Mood may be shallow, capricious or incongruous. Ambivalence and disturbance of volition may appear as inertia, negativism or stupor. Catatonia may be present. The diagnosis "schizophrenia" should not be made unless there is, or has been evident during the same illness, characteristic disturbance of thought, perception, mood, conduct, or personality—preferably in at least two of these areas. The diagnosis should not be restricted to conditions running a protracted, deteriorating, or chronic course. In addition to making the diagnosis on the criteria just given, effort should be made to specify one of the following subdivisions of schizophrenia, according to the predominant symptoms.

Includes: schizophrenia of the types described in 295.0-295.9 occurring in children

Excludes: childhood type schizophrenia (299.9)
infantile autism (299.0)

295.0 *Simple type*

A psychosis in which there is insidious development of oddities of conduct, inability to meet the demands of society, and decline in total performance. Delusions and hallucinations are not in evidence and the condition is less obviously psychotic than are the hebephrenic, catatonic and paranoid types of schizophrenia. With increasing social impoverishment vagrancy may ensue and the patient becomes self-absorbed, idle and aimless. Because the schizophrenic symptoms are not clear-cut, diagnosis of this form should be made sparingly, if at all.

Schizophrenia simplex

Excludes: latent schizophrenia (295.5)

295.1 *Hebephrenic type*

A form of schizophrenia in which affective changes are prominent, delusions and hallucinations fleeting and fragmentary, behaviour irresponsible and unpredictable and mannerisms common. The mood is shallow and inappropriate, accompanied by giggling or self-satisfied, self-absorbed smiling, or by a lofty manner, grimaces, mannerisms, pranks, hypochondriacal complaints and reiterated phrases. Thought is disorganized. There is a tendency to remain solitary, and behaviour seems empty of purpose and feeling. This form of schizophrenia usually starts between the ages of 15 and 25 years.

Hebephrenia

295.2   *Catatonic type*

Includes as an essential feature prominent psychomotor disturbances often alternating between extremes such as hyperkinesis and stupor, or automatic obedience and negativism. Constrained attitudes may be maintained for long periods: if the patient's limbs are put in some unnatural position they may be held there for some time after the external force has been removed. Severe excitement may be a striking feature of the condition. Depressive or hypomanic concomitants may be present.

Catatonic: Schizophrenic:
  agitation   catalepsy
  excitation   catatonia
  stupor   flexibilitas cerea

295.3   *Paranoid type*

The form of schizophrenia in which relatively stable delusions, which may be accompanied by hallucinations, dominate the clinical picture. The delusions are frequently of persecution but may take other forms [for example of jealousy, exalted birth, Messianic mission, or bodily change]. Hallucinations and erratic behaviour may occur; in some cases conduct is seriously disturbed from the outset, thought disorder may be gross, and affective flattening with fragmentary delusions and hallucinations may develop.

Paraphrenic schizophrenia

Excludes: paraphrenia, involutional paranoid state (297.2)
                 paranoia (297.1)

295.4   *Acute schizophrenic episode*

Schizophrenic disorders, other than those listed above, in which there is a dream-like state with slight clouding of consciousness and perplexity. External things, people and events may become charged with personal significance for the patient. There may be ideas of reference and emotional turmoil. In many such cases remission occurs within a few weeks or months, even without treatment.

Oneirophrenia   Schizophreniform:
                                                                        attack
                                                                        psychosis, confusional type

Excludes: acute forms of schizophrenia of:
                 catatonic type (295.2)
                 hebephrenic type (295.1)
                 paranoid type (295.3)
                 simple type (295.0)

295.5   *Latent schizophrenia*

It has not been possible to produce a generally acceptable description for this condition. It is not recommended for general use, but a description is provided for those who believe it to be useful: a condition of eccentric or inconsequent behaviour and anomalies of affect which give the impression of schizophrenia though no definite and characteristic schizophrenic anomalies, present or past, have been manifest.

The inclusion terms indicate that this is the best place to classify some other poorly defined varieties of schizophrenia.

Latent schizophrenic reaction
Schizophrenia:
  borderline
  prepsychotic
  prodromal

Schizophrenia:
  pseudoneurotic
  pseudopsychopathic

Excludes: schizoid personality (301.2)

295.6 *Residual schizophrenia*

A chronic form of schizophrenia in which the symptoms that persist from the acute phase have mostly lost their sharpness. Emotional response is blunted and thought disorder, even when gross, does not prevent the accomplishment of routine work.

Chronic undifferentiated schizophrenia
Restzustand (schizophrenic)
Schizophrenic residual state

295.7 *Schizoaffective type*

A psychosis in which pronounced manic or depressive features are intermingled with schizophrenic features and which tends towards remission without permanent defect, but which is prone to recur. The diagnosis should be made only when both the affective and schizophrenic symptoms are pronounced.

Cyclic schizophrenia
Mixed schizophrenic and affective psychosis
Schizoaffective psychosis
Schizophreniform psychosis, affective type

295.8 *Other*

Schizophrenia of specified type not classifiable under 295.0-295.7.

Acute (undifferentiated)
  schizophrenia

Atypical schizophrenia
Coenesthopathic schizophrenia

Excludes: infantile autism (299.0)

295.9 *Unspecified*

To be used only as a last resort.

Schizophrenia NOS
Schizophrenic reaction NOS
Schizophreniform psychosis NOS

296 Affective psychoses

Mental disorders, usually recurrent, in which there is a severe disturbance of mood [mostly compounded of depression and anxiety but also manifested as elation and excitement] which is accompanied by one or more of the following: delusions, perplexity, disturbed attitude to self, disorder of perception and behaviour; these are all in keeping with the patient's prevailing mood [as are hallucinations when they occur]. There is a strong tendency to suicide. For practical reasons, mild disorders of mood may also be included here if the symptoms match closely the descriptions given; this applies particularly to mild hypomania.

Excludes: reactive depressive psychosis (298.0)
            reactive excitation (298.1)
            neurotic depression (300.4)

296.0   *Manic-depressive psychosis, manic type*

Mental disorders characterized by states of elation or excitement out of keeping with the patient's circumstances and varying from enhanced liveliness [hypomania] to violent, almost uncontrollable excitement. Aggression and anger, flight of ideas, distractibility, impaired judgement, and grandiose ideas are common.

Hypomania NOS   Manic psychosis
Hypomanic psychosis   Manic-depressive psychosis or
Mania (monopolar) NOS   reaction:
Manic disorder   hypomanic
                                         manic

Excludes: circular type if there was a previous attack of depression
            (296.2)

296.1   *Manic-depressive psychosis, depressed type*

An affective psychosis in which there is a widespread depressed mood of gloom and wretchedness with some degree of anxiety. There is often reduced activity but there may be restlessness and agitation. There is a marked tendency to recurrence; in a few cases this may be at regular intervals.

Depressive psychosis   Manic-depressive reaction,
Endogenous depression   depressed
Involutional melancholia   Monopolar depression
                                     Psychotic depression

Excludes: circular type if previous attack was of manic type (296.3)
            depression NOS (311)

296.2   *Manic-depressive psychosis, circular type but currently manic*

An affective psychosis which has appeared in both the depressive and the manic form, either alternating or separated by an interval of normality, but in which the manic form is currently present. [The manic phase is far less frequent than the depressive].

Bipolar disorder, now manic

Excludes: brief compensatory or rebound mood swings (296.8)

296.3   *Manic-depressive psychosis, circular type but currently depressed*

Circular type (see 296.2) in which the depressive form is currently present.

Bipolar disorder, now depressed

Excludes: brief compensatory or rebound mood swings (296.8)

296.4 *Manic-depressive psychosis, circular type, mixed*

An affective psychosis in which both manic and depressive symptoms are present at the same time.

296.5 *Manic-depressive psychosis, circular type, current condition not specified*

Circular type (see 296.2) in which the current condition is not specified as either manic or depressive.

296.6 *Manic-depressive psychosis, other and unspecified*

Use this code for cases where no other information is available, except the unspecified term, manic-depressive psychosis, or for syndromes corresponding to the descriptions of depressed (296.1) or manic (296.0) types but which for other reasons cannot be classified under 296.0-296.5.

Manic-depressive psychosis:
  NOS
  mixed type

Manic-depressive:
  reaction NOS
  syndrome NOS

296.8 *Other*

Excludes: psychogenic affective psychoses (298.–)

296.9 *Unspecified*

Affective psychosis NOS
Melancholia NOS

297 Paranoid states

Excludes: acute paranoid reaction (298.3)
  alcoholic jealousy (291.5)
  paranoid schizophrenia (295.3)

297.0 *Paranoid state, simple*

A psychosis, acute or chronic, not classifiable as schizophrenia or affective psychosis, in which delusions, especially of being influenced, persecuted or treated in some special way, are the main symptoms. The delusions are of a fairly fixed, elaborate and systematized kind.

297.1 *Paranoia*

A rare chronic psychosis in which logically constructed systematized delusions have developed gradually without concomitant hallucinations or the schizophrenic type of disordered thinking. The delusions are mostly of grandeur [the paranoiac prophet or inventor], persecution or somatic abnormality.

Excludes: paranoid personality disorder (301.0)

297.2 *Paraphrenia*

Paranoid psychosis in which there are conspicuous hallucinations, often in several modalities. Affective symptoms and disordered thinking, if present, do not dominate the clinical picture and the personality is well preserved.

Involutional paranoid state
Late paraphrenia

297.3   *Induced psychosis*

Mainly delusional psychosis, usually chronic and often without florid features, which appears to have developed as a result of a close, if not dependent, relationship with another person who already has an established similar psychosis. The delusions are at least partly shared. The rare cases in which several persons are affected should also be included here.

Folie à deux   Induced paranoid disorder

297.8   *Other*

Paranoid states which, though in many ways akin to schizophrenic or affective states, cannot readily be classified under any of the preceding rubrics, nor under 298.4.

Paranoia querulans   Sensitiver Beziehungswahn

Excludes: senile paranoid state (297.2)

297.9   *Unspecified*

Paranoid:
  psychosis NOS
  reaction NOS
  state NOS

298   Other nonorganic psychoses

Categories 298.0-298.8 should be restricted to the small group of psychotic conditions that are largely or entirely attributable to a recent life experience. They should not be used for the wider range of psychoses in which environmental factors play some [but not the *major*] part in aetiology.

298.0   *Depressive type*

A depressive psychosis which can be similar in its symptoms to manic-depressive psychosis, depressed type (296.1) but is apparently provoked by saddening stress such as a bereavement, or a severe disappointment or frustration. There may be less diurnal variation of symptoms than in 296.1, and the delusions are more often understandable in the context of the life experiences. There is usually a serious disturbance of behaviour, e.g., major suicidal attempt.

Reactive depressive psychosis
Psychogenic depressive psychosis

Excludes: manic-depressive psychosis, depressed type (296.1)
            neurotic depression (300.4)

298.1   *Excitative type*

An affective psychosis similar in its symptoms to manic-depressive psychosis, manic type, but apparently provoked by emotional stress.

Excludes: manic-depressive psychosis, manic type (296.0)

298.2 *Reactive confusion*

Mental disorders with clouded consciousness, disorientation [though less marked than in organic confusion] and diminished accessibility often accompanied by excessive activity and apparently provoked by emotional stress.

Psychogenic confusion
Psychogenic twilight state

Excludes: acute confusional state (293.0)

298.3 *Acute paranoid reaction*

Paranoid states apparently provoked by some emotional stress. The stress is often misconstrued as an attack or threat. Such states are particularly prone to occur in prisoners or as acute reactions to a strange and threatening environment, e.g. in immigrants.

Bouffée délirante

Excludes: paranoid states (297.–)

298.4 *Psychogenic paranoid psychosis*

Psychogenic or reactive paranoid psychosis of any type which is more protracted than the acute reactions covered in 298.3. Where there is a diagnosis of psychogenic paranoid psychosis which does not specify "acute" this coding should be made.

Protracted reactive paranoid psychosis

298.8 *Other and unspecified reactive psychosis*

Hysterical psychosis   Psychogenic stupor
Psychogenic psychosis NOS

298.9 *Unspecified psychosis*

To be used only as a last resort, when no other term can be used.

Psychosis NOS

299   Psychoses with origin specific to childhood

This category should be used only for psychoses which always begin before puberty. Adult-type psychoses such as schizophrenia or manic-depressive psychoses when occurring in childhood should be coded elsewhere under the appropriate heading—i.e., 295 and 296 for the examples given.

299.0 *Infantile autism*

A syndrome present from birth or beginning almost invariably in the first 30 months. Responses to auditory and sometimes to visual stimuli are abnormal and there are usually severe problems in the understanding of spoken language. Speech is delayed and, if it develops, is characterized by echolalia, the reversal of pronouns, immature grammatical structure and inability to use abstract terms. There is generally an impairment in the social use of both verbal and gestural language. Problems in social relationships are most severe before the age of five years and include an impairment in the development of eye-to-eye gaze, social attachments, and cooperative play. Ritualistic behaviour is usual and may include abnormal routines, resistance to change, attachment to odd objects and stereotyped patterns of play. The capacity for abstract or symbolic thought and for imaginative play is diminished. Intelligence ranges from severely subnormal to normal or above. Performance is usually better on tasks involving rote memory or visuospatial skills than on those requiring symbolic or linguistic skills.

Childhood autism   Kanner's syndrome
Infantile psychosis

Excludes: disintegrative psychosis (299.1)
            Heller's syndrome (299.1)
            schizophrenic syndrome of childhood (299.9)

299.1   *Disintegrative psychosis*

A disorder in which normal or near-normal development for the first few years is followed by a loss of social skills and of speech, together with a severe disorder of emotions, behaviour and relationships. Usually this loss of speech and of social competence takes place over a period of a few months and is accompanied by the emergence of overactivity and of stereotypies. In most cases there is intellectual impairment, but this is not a necessary part of the disorder. The condition may follow overt brain disease—such as measles encephalitis—but it may also occur in the absence of any known organic brain disease or damage. Use additional code to identify any associated neurological disorder.

Heller's syndrome

Excludes: infantile autism (299.0)
            schizophrenic syndrome of childhood (299.9)

299.8   *Other*

A variety of atypical infantile psychoses which may show some, but not all, of the features of infantile autism. Symptoms may include stereotyped repetitive movements, hyperkinesis, self-injury, retarded speech development, echolalia and impaired social relationships. Such disorders may occur in children of any level of intelligence but are particularly common in those with mental retardation.

Atypical childhood psychosis

Excludes: simple stereotypies without psychotic disturbance (307.3)

299.9   *Unspecified*

Child psychosis NOS
Schizophrenia, childhood type NOS
Schizophrenic syndrome of childhood NOS

Excludes: schizophrenia of adult type occurring in childhood (295.0-
            295.8)

NEUROTIC DISORDERS, PERSONALITY DISORDERS AND OTHER NONPSYCHOTIC MENTAL DISORDERS (300-316)

300 Neurotic disorders

The distinction between neurosis and psychosis is difficult and remains subject to debate. However, it has been retained in view of its wide use.

Neurotic disorders are mental disorders without any demonstrable organic basis in which the patient may have considerable insight and has unimpaired reality testing, in that he usually does not confuse his morbid subjective experiences and fantasies with external reality. Behaviour may be greatly affected although usually remaining within socially acceptable limits, but personality is not disorganized. The principal manifestations include excessive anxiety, hysterical symptoms, phobias, obsessional and compulsive symptoms, and depression.

300.0 *Anxiety states*

Various combinations of physical and mental manifestations of anxiety, not attributable to real danger and occurring either in attacks or as a persisting state. The anxiety is usually diffuse and may extend to panic. Other neurotic features such as obsessional or hysterical symptoms may be present but do not dominate the clinical picture.

Anxiety:
  neurosis
  reaction
  state (neurotic)

Panic:
  attack
  disorder
  state

Excludes: neurasthenia (300.5)
  psychophysiological disorders (306.–)

300.1 *Hysteria*

Mental disorders in which motives, of which the patient seems unaware, produce either a restriction of the field of consciousness or disturbances of motor or sensory function which may seem to have psychological advantage or symbolic value. It may be characterized by conversion phenomena or dissociative phenomena. In the conversion form the chief or only symptoms consist of psychogenic disturbance of function in some part of the body, e.g., paralysis, tremor, blindness, deafness, seizures. In the dissociative variety, the most prominent feature is a narrowing of the field of consciousness which seems to serve an unconscious purpose and is commonly accompanied or followed by a selective amnesia. There may be dramatic but essentially superficial changes of personality sometimes taking the form of a fugue [wandering state]. Behaviour may mimic psychosis or, rather, the patient's idea of psychosis.

Astasia-abasia, hysterical
Compensation neurosis
Conversion hysteria
Conversion reaction

Dissociative reaction or state
Ganser's syndrome, hysterical
Hysteria NOS
Multiple personality

Excludes: adjustment reaction (309.–)
  anorexia nervosa (307.1)
  gross stress reaction (308.–)
  hysterical personality (301.5)
  psychophysiological disorders (306.–)

300.2   *Phobic state*

Neurotic states with abnormally intense dread of certain objects or specific situations which would not normally have that effect. If the anxiety tends to spread from a specified situation or object to a wider range of circumstances, it becomes akin to or identical with anxiety state, and should be classified as such (300.0).

Agoraphobia   Claustrophobia
Animal phobias   Phobia NOS
Anxiety-hysteria

Excludes: anxiety state (300.0)
            obsessional phobias (300.3)

300.3   *Obsessive-compulsive disorders*

States in which the outstanding symptom is a feeling of subjective compulsion—which must be resisted—to carry out some action, to dwell on an idea, to recall an experience, or to ruminate on an abstract topic. Unwanted thoughts which intrude, the insistency of words or ideas, ruminations or trains of thought are perceived by the patient to be inappropriate or nonsensical. The obsessional urge or idea is recognized as alien to the personality but as coming from within the self. Obsessional actions may be quasi-ritual performances designed to relieve anxiety e.g., washing the hands to cope with contamination. Attempts to dispel the unwelcome thoughts or urges may lead to a severe inner struggle, with intense anxiety.

Anankastic neurosis
Compulsive neurosis

Excludes: obsessive-compulsive symptoms occurring in:
            endogenous depression (296.1)
            schizophrenia (295.–)
            organic states, e.g., encephalitis

300.4   *Neurotic depression*

A neurotic disorder characterized by disproportionate depression which has usually recognizably ensued on a distressing experience; it does not include among its features delusions or hallucinations, and there is often preoccupation with the psychic trauma which preceded the illness, e.g., loss of a cherished person or possession. Anxiety is also frequently present and mixed states of anxiety and depression should be included here. The distinction between depressive neurosis and psychosis should be made not only upon the degree of depression but also on the presence or absence of other neurotic and psychotic characteristics and upon the degree of disturbance of the patient's behaviour.

Anxiety depression   Neurotic depressive state
Depressive reaction   Reactive depression

Excludes: adjustment reaction with depressive symptoms (309.0)
            depression NOS (311)
            manic-depressive psychosis, depressed type (296.1)
            reactive depressive psychosis (298.0)

300.5 *Neurasthenia*

A neurotic disorder characterized by fatigue, irritability, headache, depression, insomnia, difficulty in concentration, and lack of capacity for enjoyment [anhedonia]. It may follow or accompany an infection or exhaustion, or arise from continued emotional stress. If neurasthenia is associated with a physical disorder, the latter should also be coded.

Nervous debility

Excludes: anxiety state (300.0)
 neurotic depression (300.4)
 psychophysiological disorders (306.–)
 specific nonpsychotic mental disorders following organic brain damage (310.–)

300.6 *Depersonalization syndrome*

A neurotic disorder with an unpleasant state of disturbed perception in which external objects or parts of one's own body are experienced as changed in their quality, unreal, remote or automatized. The patient is aware of the subjective nature of the change he experiences. Depersonalization may occur as a feature of several mental disorders including depression, obsessional neurosis, anxiety and schizophrenia; in that case the condition should not be classified here but in the corresponding major category.

Derealization (neurotic)

300.7 *Hypochondriasis*

A neurotic disorder in which the conspicuous features are excessive concern with one's health in general or the integrity and functioning of some part of one's body, or, less frequently, one's mind. It is usually associated with anxiety and depression. It may occur as a feature of severe mental disorder and in that case should not be classified here but in the corresponding major category.

Excludes: hysteria (300.1)
 manic-depressive psychosis, depressed type (296.1)
 neurasthenia (300.5)
 obsessional disorder (300.3)
 schizophrenia (295.–)

300.8 *Other neurotic disorders*

Neurotic disorders not classified elsewhere, e.g., occupational neurosis. Patients with mixed neuroses should not be classified in this category but according to the most prominent symptoms they display.

Briquet's disorder
Occupational neurosis, including writer's cramp
Psychasthenia
Psychasthenic neurosis

300.9 *Unspecified*

To be used only as a last resort.

Neurosis NOS   Psychoneurosis NOS

301   Personality disorders

Deeply ingrained maladaptive patterns of behaviour generally recognizable by the time of adolescence or earlier and continuing throughout most of adult life, although often becoming less obvious in middle or old age. The personality is abnormal either in the balance of its components, their quality and expression or in its total aspect. Because of this deviation or psychopathy the patient suffers or others have to suffer and there is an adverse effect upon the individual or on society. It includes what is sometimes called psychopathic personality, but if this is determined primarily by malfunctioning of the brain, it should not be classified here but as one of the nonpsychotic organic brain syndromes (310). When the patient exhibits an anomaly of personality directly related to his neurosis or psychosis, e.g., schizoid personality and schizophrenia or anankastic personality and obsessive compulsive neurosis, the relevant neurosis or psychosis which is in evidence should be diagnosed in addition.

Character neurosis

301.0   *Paranoid personality disorder*

Personality disorder in which there is excessive sensitiveness to setbacks or to what are taken to be humiliations and rebuffs, a tendency to distort experience by misconstruing the neutral or friendly actions of others as hostile or contemptuous, and a combative and tenacious sense of personal rights. There may be a proneness to jealousy or excessive self-importance. Such persons may feel helplessly humiliated and put upon; others, likewise excessively sensitive, are agressive and insistent. In all cases there is excessive self-reference.

Fanatic personality   Paranoid personality (disorder)
Paranoid traits

Excludes: acute paranoid reaction (298.3)
            alcoholic paranoia (291.5)
            paranoid schizophrenia (295.3)
            paranoid states (297.–)

301.1   *Affective personality disorder*

Personality disorder characterized by lifelong predominance of a pronounced mood which may be persistently depressive, persistently elated, or alternately one then the other. During periods of elation there is unshakeable optimism and an enhanced zest for life and activity, whereas periods of depression are marked by worry, pessimism, low output of energy and a sense of futility.

Cycloid personality   Depressive personality
Cyclothymic personality

Excludes: affective psychoses (296.–)
            cyclothymia (296.2–296.5)
            neurasthenia (300.5)
            neurotic depression (300.4)

301.2   *Schizoid personality disorder*

Personality disorder in which there is withdrawal from affectional, social and other contacts with autistic preference for fantasy and introspective reserve. Behaviour may be slightly eccentric or indicate avoidance of competitive situations. Apparent coolness and detachment may mask an incapacity to express feeling.

Excludes: schizophrenia (295.–)

301.3 *Explosive personality disorder*

Personality disorder characterized by instability of mood with liability to intemperate outbursts of anger, hate, violence or affection. Aggression may be expressed in words or in physical violence. The outbursts cannot readily be controlled by the affected persons, who are not otherwise prone to antisocial behaviour.

Aggressive:
  personality
  reaction
Aggressiveness

Emotional instability (excessive)
Pathological emotionality
Quarrelsomeness

Excludes: dyssocial personality (301.7)
          hysterical neurosis (300.1)

301.4 *Anankastic personality disorder*

Personality disorder characterized by feelings of personal insecurity, doubt and incompleteness leading to excessive conscientiousness, checking, stubborness and caution. There may be insistent and unwelcome thoughts or impulses which do not attain the severity of an obsessional neurosis. There is perfectionism and meticulous accuracy and a need to check repeatedly in an attempt to ensure this. Rigidity and excessive doubt may be conspicuous.

Compulsive personality   Obsessional personality

Excludes: obsessive-compulsive disorder (300.3)
          phobic state (300.2)

301.5 *Hysterical personality disorder*

Personality disorder characterized by shallow, labile affectivity, dependence on others, craving for appreciation and attention, suggestibility and theatricality. There is often sexual immaturity, e.g., frigidity and over-responsiveness to stimuli. Under stress hysterical symptoms [neurosis] may develop.

Histrionic personality   Psychoinfantile personality

Excludes: hysterical neurosis (300.1)

301.6 *Asthenic personality disorder*

Personality disorder characterized by passive compliance with the wishes of elders and others and a weak inadequate response to the demands of daily life. Lack of vigour may show itself in the intellectual or emotional spheres; there is little capacity for enjoyment.

Dependent personality   Passive personality
Inadequate personality

Excludes: neurasthenia (300.5)

301.7 *Personality disorder with predominantly sociopathic or asocial manifestation*

Personality disorder characterized by disregard for social obligations, lack of feeling for others, and impetuous violence or callous unconcern. There is a gross disparity between behaviour and the prevailing social norms. Behaviour is not readily modifiable by experience, including punishment. People with this personality are often affectively cold and may be abnormally aggressive or irresponsible. Their tolerance to frustration is low; they blame others or offer plausible rationalizations for the behaviour which brings them into conflict with society.

Amoral personality   Asocial personality
Antisocial personality

Excludes: disturbance of conduct without specifiable personality disorder (312.–)
           explosive personality (301.3)

301.8 *Other personality disorders*

Personality: Personality:
   eccentric   immature
   "haltlose" type   passive-aggressive
                                                   psychoneurotic

Excludes: psychoinfantile personality (301.5)

301.9 *Unspecified*

Pathological personality NOS   Psychopathic:
Personality disorder NOS   constitutional state
                                                   personality (disorder)

302   Sexual deviations and disorders

Abnormal sexual inclinations or behaviour which are part of a referral problem. The limits and features of normal sexual inclination and behaviour have not been stated absolutely in different societies and cultures but are broadly such as serve approved social and biological purposes. The sexual activity of affected persons is directed primarily either towards people not of the opposite sex, or towards sexual acts not associated with coitus normally, or towards coitus performed under abnormal circumstances. If the anomalous behaviour becomes manifest only during psychosis or other mental illness the condition should be classified under the major illness. It is common for more than one anomaly to occur together in the same individual; in that case the predominant deviation is classified. It is preferable not to include in this category individuals who perform deviant sexual acts when normal sexual outlets are not available to them.

302.0 *Homosexuality*

Exclusive or predominant sexual attraction for persons of the same sex with or without physical relationship. Code homosexuality here whether or not it is considered as a mental disorder.

Lesbianism

Excludes: homosexual paedophilia (302.2)

302.1 *Bestiality*

Sexual or anal intercourse with animals.

302.2 *Paedophilia*

Sexual deviations in which an adult engages in sexual activity with a child of the same or opposite sex.

302.3 *Transvestism*

Sexual deviation in which sexual pleasure is derived from dressing in clothes of the opposite sex. There is no consistent attempt to take on the identity or behaviour of the opposite sex.

Excludes: trans-sexualism (302.5)

302.4 *Exhibitionism*

Sexual deviation in which the main sexual pleasure and gratification is derived from exposure of the genitals to a person of the opposite sex.

302.5 *Trans-sexualism*

Sexual deviation centred around fixed beliefs that the overt bodily sex is wrong. The resulting behaviour is directed towards either changing the sexual organs by operation, or completely concealing the bodily sex by adopting both the dress and behaviour of the opposite sex.

Excludes: transvestism (302.3)

302.6 *Disorders of psychosexual identity*

Behaviour occurring in preadolescents of immature psychosexuality which is similar to that shown in the sexual deviations described under transvestism (302.3) and trans-sexualism (302.5). Cross-dressing is intermittent, although it may be frequent, and identification with the behaviour and appearance of the opposite sex is not yet fixed. The commonest form is feminism in boys.

Gender-role disorder

Excludes: homosexuality (302.0)
            trans-sexualism (302.5)
            transvestism (302.3)

302.7 *Frigidity and impotence*

Frigidity—dislike of or aversion to sexual intercourse, of psychological origin, of sufficient intensity to lead, if not to active avoidance, to marked anxiety, discomfort or pain when normal sexual intercourse takes place. Less severe degrees of this disorder that also give rise to consultation should also be coded here.

Impotence—sustained inability, due to psychological causes, to maintain an erection which will allow normal heterosexual penetration and ejaculation to take place.

Dyspareunia, psychogenic

Excludes: impotence of organic origin
            normal transient symptoms from ruptured hymen
            transient or occasional failures of erection due to fatigue,
                anxiety, alcohol or drugs

302.8 *Other*

Fetishism   Sadism
Masochism

302.9 *Unspecified*

303   Alcohol dependence syndrome

A state, psychic and usually also physical, resulting from taking alcohol, characterized by behavioural and other responses that always include a compulsion to take alcohol on a continuous or periodic basis in order to experience its psychic effects, and sometimes to avoid the discomfort of its absence; tolerance may or may not be present. A person may be dependent on alcohol and other drugs; if so also make the appropriate 304 coding. If dependence is associated with alcoholic psychosis or with physical complications, *both* should be coded.

Acute drunkenness in alcoholism   Dipsomania
Chronic alcoholism

Excludes: alcoholic psychoses (291.–)
            drunkenness NOS (305.0)
            physical complications of alcohol, such as:
              cirrhosis of liver (571.2)
              epilepsy (345.–)
              gastritis (535.3)

304   Drug dependence

A state, psychic and sometimes also physical, resulting from taking a drug, characterized by behavioural and other responses that always include a compulsion to take a drug on a continuous or periodic basis in order to experience its psychic effects, and sometimes to avoid the discomfort of its absence. Tolerance may or may not be present. A person may be dependent on more than one drug.

Excludes: nondependent abuse of drugs (305.–)

304.0   *Morphine type*

Heroin   Opium alkaloids and their deriva-
Methadone   tives
Opium   Synthetics with morphine-like
                                  effects

304.1   *Barbiturate type*

Barbiturates
Nonbarbiturate sedatives and tranquillizers with a similar effect:
  chlordiazepoxide
  diazepam
  glutethimide
  meprobamate

304.2   *Cocaine*

Coca leaves and derivatives

304.3   *Cannabis*

Hemp   Marijuana
Hashish

304.4 *Amphetamine type and other psychostimulants*

Phenmetrazine   Methylphenidate

304.5 *Hallucinogens*

LSD and derivatives   Psilocybin
Mescaline

304.6 *Other*

Absinthe addiction   Glue sniffing

Excludes: tobacco dependence (305.1)

304.7 *Combinations of morphine type drug with any other*

304.8 *Combinations excluding morphine type drug*

304.9 *Unspecified*

Drug addiction NOS   Drug dependence NOS

305   Nondependent abuse of drugs

Includes cases where a person, for whom no other diagnosis is possible, has come under medical care because of the maladaptive effect of a drug on which he is not dependent (as defined in 304.–) and that he has taken on his own initiative to the detriment of his health or social functioning. When drug abuse is secondary to a psychiatric disorder, code the disorder.

Excludes: alcohol dependence syndrome (303)
          drug dependence (304.–)
          drug withdrawal syndrome (292.0)
          poisoning by drugs or medicaments (960-979)

305.0 *Alcohol*

Cases of acute intoxication or "hangover" effects.

Drunkenness NOS   "Hangover" (alcohol)
Excessive drinking of alcohol NOS   Inebriety NOS

Excludes: alcoholic psychoses (291.–)
          physical complications of alcohol, such as:
             cirrhosis of liver (571.2)
             epilepsy (345.–)
             gastritis (535.3)

305.1 *Tobacco*

Cases in which tobacco is used to the detriment of a person's health or social functioning or in which there is tobacco dependence. Dependence is included here rather than under 304.– because tobacco differs from other drugs of dependence in its psychotoxic effects.

Tobacco dependence

305.2 *Cannabis*

305.3   *Hallucinogens*

Cases of acute intoxication or "bad trips".

LSD reaction

305.4   *Barbiturates and tranquillizers*

Cases where a person has taken the drug to the detriment of his health or social functioning, in doses above or for periods beyond those normally regarded as therapeutic.

305.5   *Morphine type*

305.6   *Cocaine type*

305.7   *Amphetamine type*

305.8   *Antidepressants*

305.9   *Other, mixed or unspecified*

"Laxative habit"   Nonprescribed use of drugs or
Misuse of drugs NOS   patent medicinals

306   Physiological malfunction arising from mental factors

A variety of physical symptoms or types of physiological malfunction of mental origin, not involving tissue damage and usually mediated through the autonomic nervous system. The disorders are grouped according to body system. Codes 306.0-306.9 should not be used if the physical symptom is secondary to a psychiatric disorder classifiable elsewhere. If tissue damage is involved, code under 316.

Excludes: hysteria (300.1)
            psychic factors associated with physical conditions involving
               tissue damage classified elsewhere (316)
            specific nonpsychotic mental disorders following organic
               brain damage (310.–)

306.0   *Musculoskeletal*

Psychogenic torticollis

Excludes: Gilles de la Tourette's syndrome (307.2)
            tics (307.2)

306.1   *Respiratory*

Air hunger   Psychogenic cough
Hiccough (psychogenic)   Yawning
Hyperventilation

Excludes: psychogenic asthma (316 and 493.9)

306.2   *Cardiovascular*

Cardiac neurosis   Neurocirculatory asthenia
Cardiovascular neurosis   Psychogenic cardiovascular
                                           disorder

Excludes: psychogenic paroxysmal tachycardia (316 and 427.9)

306.3   *Skin*

Psychogenic pruritus

Excludes: psychogenic:
        alopecia (316 and 704.0)
        dermatitis (316 and 692.–)
        eczema (316 and 691.9 or 692.–)
        urticaria (316 and 708.–)

306.4   *Gastrointestinal*

Aerophagy   Cyclical vomiting, psychogenic

Excludes: cyclical vomiting NOS (536.2)
        mucous colitis (316 and 564.1)
        psychogenic:
           cardiospasm (316 and 530.0)
           duodenal ulcer (316 and 532.–)
           gastric ulcer (316 and 531.–)
           peptic ulcer (316 and 533.–)

306.5   *Genitourinary*

Psychogenic dysmenorrhoea

Excludes: dyspareunia (302.7)
        enuresis (307.6)
        frigidity (302.7)
        impotence (302.7)

306.6   *Endocrine*

306.7   *Organs of special sense*

Excludes: hysterical blindness or deafness (300.1)

306.8   *Other*

Teeth-grinding

306.9   *Unspecified*

Psychophysiologic disorder NOS   Psychosomatic disorder NOS

307   Special symptoms or syndromes not elsewhere classified

Conditions in which an outstanding symptom or group of symptoms is not manifestly part of a more fundamental classifiable condition.

Excludes: when due to mental disorders classified elsewhere
        when of organic origin

307.0   *Stammering and stuttering*

Disorders in the rhythm of speech, in which the individual knows precisely what he wishes to say, but at the time is unable to say it because of an involuntary, repetitive prolongation or cessation of a sound.

Excludes: dysphasia (784.5)
         lisping or lalling (307.9)
         retarded development of speech (315.3)

307.1   *Anorexia nervosa*

A disorder in which the main features are persistent active refusal to eat and marked loss of weight.   The level of activity and alertness is characteristically high in relation to the degree of emaciation.   Typically the disorder begins in teenage girls but it may sometimes begin before puberty and rarely it occurs in males.   Amenorrhoea is usual and there may be a variety of other physiological changes including slow pulse and respiration, low body temperature and dependent oedema.   Unusual eating habits and attitudes toward food are typical and sometimes starvation follows or alternates with periods of overeating.   The accompanying psychiatric symptoms are diverse.

Excludes: eating disturbance NOS (307.5)
         loss of appetite (783.0)
         of nonorganic origin (307.5)

307.2   *Tics*

Disorders of no known organic origin in which the outstanding feature consists of quick, involuntary, apparently purposeless, and frequently repeated movements which are not due to any neurological condition.   Any part of the body may be involved but the face is most frequently affected.   Only one form of tic may be present, or there may be a combination of tics which are carried out simultaneously, alternatively or consecutively.   Gilles de la Tourette's syndrome refers to a rare disorder occurring in individuals of any level of intelligence in which facial tics and tic-like throat noises become more marked and more generalized and in which later, whole words or short sentences [often with an obscene content] are ejaculated spasmodically and involuntarily.   There is some overlap with other varieties of tic.

Excludes: nail-biting or thumb-sucking (307.9)
         stereotypies occurring in isolation (307.3)
         tics of organic origin (333.3)

307.3   *Stereotyped repetitive movements*

Disorders in which voluntary repetitive stereotyped movements, which are not due to any psychiatric or neurological condition, constitute the main feature.   Includes head-banging, spasmus nutans, rocking, twirling, finger-flicking mannerisms and eye poking. Such movements are particularly common in cases of mental retardation with sensory impairment or with environmental monotony.

Stereotypies NOS

Excludes: tics:
         NOS (307.2)
         of organic origin (333.3)

307.4 *Specific disorders of sleep*

This category should only be used when a more precise medical or psychiatric diagnosis cannot be made.

Hypersomnia
Insomnia
Inversion of sleep rhythm
Nightmares
Night terrors
Sleepwalking
} of nonorganic origin

Excludes: narcolepsy (347.0)
when of unspecified cause (780.5)

307.5 *Other and unspecified disorders of eating*

This category should only be used when a more precise medical or psychiatric diagnosis cannot be made.

Infantile feeding disturbances
Loss of appetite
Overeating
Pica
} of nonorganic origin

Psychogenic vomiting

Excludes: anorexia:
nervosa (307.1)
of unspecified cause (783.0)
overeating of unspecified cause (783.6)
vomiting:
NOS (787.0)
cyclical (536.2)
psychogenic (306.4)

307.6 *Enuresis*

A disorder in which the main manifestation is a persistent involuntary voiding of urine by day or night which is considered abnormal for the age of the individual. Sometimes the child will have failed to gain bladder control and in other cases he will have gained control and then lost it. Episodic or fluctuating enuresis should be included. The disorder would not usually be diagnosed under the age of four years.

Enuresis (primary) (secondary) of nonorganic origin

Excludes: enuresis of unspecified cause (788.3)

307.7 *Encopresis*

A disorder in which the main manifestation is the persistent voluntary or involuntary passage of formed motions of normal or near-normal consistency into places not intended for that purpose in the individual's own sociocultural setting. Sometimes the child has failed to gain bowel control, and sometimes he has gained control but then later again became encopretic. There may be a variety of associated psychiatric symptoms and there may be smearing of faeces. The condition would not usually be diagnosed under the age of four years.

Encopresis (continuous) (discontinuous) of nonorganic origin

Excludes: encopresis of unspecified cause (787.6)

307.8 *Psychalgia*

Cases in which there are pains of mental origin, e.g., headache or backache, when a more precise medical or psychiatric diagnosis cannot be made.

Tension headache   Psychogenic backache

Excludes: migraine (346.–)
                 pains not specifically attributable to a psychological cause
                    (in):
                    back (724.5)
                    headache (784.0)
                    joint (719.4)
                    limb (729.5)
                    lumbago (724.2)
                    rheumatic (729.0)

307.9 *Other and unspecified*

The use of this category should be discouraged. Most of the items listed in the inclusion terms are not indicative of psychiatric disorder and are included only because such terms may sometimes still appear as diagnoses.

Hair plucking   Masturbation
Lalling   Nail-biting
Lisping   Thumb-sucking

308   Acute reaction to stress

Very transient disorders of any severity and nature which occur in individuals without any apparent mental disorder in response to exceptional physical or mental stress, such as natural catastrophe or battle, and which usually subside within hours or days.

Catastrophic stress   Exhaustion delirium
Combat fatigue

Excludes: adjustment reaction (309.–)

308.0 *Predominant disturbance of emotions*

Panic states, excitability, fear, depressions and anxiety fulfilling the above criteria.

308.1 *Predominant disturbance of consciousness*

Fugues fulfilling the above criteria.

308.2 *Predominant psychomotor disturbance*

Agitation states, stupor fulfilling the above criteria.

308.3 *Other*

Acute situational disturbance

308.4 *Mixed*

Many gross stress reactions include several elements but whenever possible a specific coding under .0, .1, .2 or .3 should be made according to the *preponderant* type of disturbance. The category of mixed disorders should only be used when there is such an admixture that this cannot be done.

308.9   *Unspecified*

309   Adjustment reaction

Mild or transient disorders lasting longer than acute stress reactions (308.–) which occur in individuals of any age without any apparent pre-existing mental disorder. Such disorders are often relatively circumscribed or situation-specific, are generally reversible, and usually last only a few months. They are usually closely related in time and content to stresses such as bereavement, migration or separation experiences. Reactions to major stress that last longer than a few days are also included here. In children such disorders are associated with no significant distortion of development.

Excludes: acute reaction to major stress (308.–)
            neurotic disorders (300.–)

309.0   *Brief depressive reaction*

States of depression, not specifiable as manic-depressive, psychotic or neurotic, generally transient, in which the depressive symptoms are usually closely related in time and content to some stressful event.

Grief reaction

Excludes: affective psychoses (296.–)
            neurotic depression (300.4)
            prolonged depressive reaction (309.1)
            psychogenic depressive psychosis (298.0)

309.1   *Prolonged depressive reaction*

States of depression, not specifiable as manic-depressive, psychotic or neurotic, generally long-lasting; usually developing in association with prolonged exposure to a stressful situation.

Excludes: affective psychoses (296.–)
            brief depressive reaction (309.0)
            neurotic depression (300.4)
            psychogenic depressive psychosis (298.0)

309.2   *With predominant disturbance of other emotions*

States, fulfilling the general criteria for adjustment reaction, in which the main symptoms are emotional in type [anxiety, fear, worry, etc.] but not specifically depressive.

Abnormal separation anxiety   Culture shock

309.3   *With predominant disturbance of conduct*

Mild or transient disorders, fulfilling the general criteria for adjustment reaction, in which the main disturbance predominantly involves a disturbance of conduct. For example, an adolescent grief reaction resulting in aggressive or antisocial disorder would be included here.

Excludes: disturbance of conduct NOS (312.–)
            dyssocial behaviour without manifest psychiatric disorder (V71.0)
            personality disorder with predominantly sociopathic or asocial manifestations (301.7)

309.4   *With mixed disturbance of emotions and conduct*

Disorders fulfilling the general definition in which both emotional disturbance and disturbance of conduct are prominent features.

309.8   *Other*

Adjustment reaction with elective mutism
Hospitalism in children NOS

309.9   *Unspecified*

Adjustment reaction NOS   Adaptation reaction NOS

310   Specific nonpsychotic mental disorders following organic brain damage

Note: This category should be used only for conditions where the *form* of the disorder is determined by the brain pathology.

Excludes: neuroses, personality disorders or other nonpsychotic conditions occurring in a form similar to that seen with functional disorders but in association with a physical condition; code to 300.–, 301.–, etc., and use additional code to identify the physical condition

310.0   *Frontal lobe syndrome*

Changes in behaviour following damage to the frontal areas of the brain or following interference with the connections of those areas.   There is a general diminution of self-control, foresight, creativity and spontaneity, which may be manifest as increased irritability, selfishness, restlessness and lack of concern for others.   Conscientiousness and powers of concentration are often diminished, but measurable deterioration of intellect or memory is not necessarily present.   The overall picture is often one of emotional dullness, lack of drive and slowness; but, particularly in persons previously with energetic, restless or aggressive characteristics, there may be a change towards impulsiveness, boastfulness, temper outbursts, silly fatuous humour, and the development of unrealistic ambitions; the direction of change usually depends upon the previous personality.   A considerable degree of recovery is possible and may continue over the course of several years.

Lobotomy syndrome
Postleucotomy syndrome (state)

Excludes: postcontusional syndrome (310.2)

310.1   *Cognitive or personality change of other type*

Chronic, mild states of memory disturbance and intellectual deterioration, often accompanied by increased irritability, querulousness, lassitude and complaints of physical weakness.   These states are often associated with old age, and may precede more severe states due to brain damage classifiable under dementia of any type (290.–, and 294.–) or any condition in 293.– (Transient organic psychotic conditions).

Mild memory disturbance
Organic psychosyndrome of nonpsychotic severity

310.2 *Postconcussional syndrome*

States occurring after generalized contusion of the brain, in which the symptom picture may resemble that of the frontal lobe syndrome (310.0) or that of any of the neurotic disorders (300.0-300.9), but in which in addition, headache, giddiness, fatigue, insomnia and a subjective feeling of impaired intellectual ability are usually prominent. Mood may fluctuate, and quite ordinary stress may produce exaggerated fear and apprehension. There may be marked intolerance of mental and physical exertion, undue sensitivity to noise, and hypochondriacal preoccupation. The symptoms are more common in persons who have previously suffered from neurotic or personality disorders, or when there is a possibility of compensation. This syndrome is particularly associated with the closed type of head injury when signs of localized brain damage are slight or absent, but it may also occur in other conditions.

Postcontusional syndrome (encephalopathy)
Status post commotio cerebri
Post-traumatic brain syndrome, nonpsychotic

Excludes: frontal lobe syndrome (310.0)
        postencephalitic syndrome (310.8)
        any organic psychotic conditions following head injury (290.– to 294.0)

310.8 *Other*

Include here disorders resembling the postcontusional syndrome (310.2), associated with infective or other diseases of the brain or surrounding tissues.

Other focal (partial) organic psychosyndromes

310.9 *Unspecified*

311 Depressive disorder, not elsewhere classified

States of depression, usually of moderate but occasionally of marked intensity, which have no specifically manic-depressive or other psychotic depressive features and which do not appear to be associated with stressful events or other features specified under neurotic depression.

Depressive disorder NOS   Depression NOS
Depressive state NOS

Excludes: acute reaction to major stress with depressive symptoms (308.0)
        affective personality disorder (301.1)
        affective psychoses (296.–)
        brief depressive reaction (309.0)
        disturbance of emotions specific to childhood and adolescence, with misery and unhappiness (313.1)
        mixed adjustment reaction with depressive symptoms (309.4)
        neurotic depression (300.4)
        prolonged depressive adjustment reaction (309.1)
        psychogenic depressive psychosis (298.0)

312   Disturbance of conduct not elsewhere classified

Disorders mainly involving aggressive and destructive behaviour and disorders involving delinquency. It should be used for abnormal behaviour, in individuals of any age, which gives rise to social disapproval but which is not part of any other psychiatric condition. Minor emotional disturbances may also be present. To be included, the behaviour—as judged by its frequency, severity and type of associations with other symptoms—must be abnormal in its context. Disturbances of conduct are distinguished from an adjustment reaction by a longer duration and by a lack of close relationship in time and content to some stress. They differ from a personality disorder by the absence of deeply ingrained maladapative patterns of behaviour present from adolescence or earlier.

Excludes: adjustment reaction with disturbance of conduct (309.3)
                  drug dependence (304.–)
                  dyssocial behaviour without manifest psychiatric disorder
                  (V71.0)
                  personality disorder with predominantly sociopathic or
                  asocial manifestations (301.7)
                  sexual deviations (302.–)

312.0   *Unsocialized disturbance of conduct*

Disorders characterized by behaviours such as defiance, disobedience, quarrelsomeness, aggression, destructive behaviour, tantrums, solitary stealing, lying, teasing, bullying and disturbed relationships with others. The defiance may sometimes take the form of sexual misconduct.

Unsocialized aggressive disorder

312.1   *Socialized disturbance of conduct*

Disorders in individuals who have acquired the values or behaviour of a delinquent peer group to whom they are loyal and with whom they characteristically steal, play truant, and stay out late at night. There may also be promiscuity.

Group delinquency

Excludes: gang activity without manifest psychiatric disorder (V71.0)

312.2   *Compulsive conduct disorder*

Disorder of conduct or delinquent act which is specifically compulsive in origin.

Kleptomania

312.3   *Mixed disturbance of conduct and emotions*

Disorders involving behaviours listed for 312.0 and 312.1 but in which there is also *considerable* emotional disturbance as shown for example by anxiety, misery or obsessive manifestations.

Neurotic delinquency

Excludes: compulsive conduct disorder (312.2)

312.8   *Other*

312.9   *Unspecified*

313   Disturbance of emotions specific to childhood and adolescence

Less well differentiated emotional disorders characteristic of the childhood period. Where the emotional disorder takes the form of a neurotic disorder described under 300.–, the appropriate 300.– coding should be made. This category differs from category 308.– in terms of longer duration and by the lack of close relationship in time and content to some stress.

Excludes: adjustment reaction (309.–)
              masturbation, nail-biting, thumb-sucking and other isolated symptoms (307.–)

313.0   *With anxiety and fearfulness*

Ill-defined emotional disorders characteristic of childhood in which the main symptoms involve anxiety and fearfulness. Many cases of school refusal or elective mutism might be included here.

Overanxious reaction of childhood or adolescence

Excludes: abnormal separation anxiety (309.2)
              anxiety states (300.0)
              hospitalism in children (309.8)
              phobic state (300.2)

313.1   *With misery and unhappiness*

Emotional disorders characteristic of childhood in which the main symptoms involve misery and unhappiness. There may also be eating and sleep disturbances.

Excludes: depressive neurosis (300.4)

313.2   *With sensitivity, shyness and social withdrawal*

Emotional disorders characteristic of childhood in which the main symptoms involve sensitivity, shyness, or social withdrawal. Some cases of elective mutism might be included here.

Withdrawing reaction of childhood or adolescence

Excludes: infantile autism (299.0)
              schizoid personality (301.2)
              schizophrenia (295.–)

313.3   *Relationship problems*

Emotional disorders characteristic of childhood in which the main symptoms involve relationship problems.

Sibling jealousy

Excludes: relationship problems associated with aggression, destruction or other forms of conduct disturbance (312.–)

313.8   *Other or mixed*

Many emotional disorders of childhood include several elements but whenever possible a specific coding under .0, .1, .2 or .3 should be made according to the *preponderant* type of disturbance. The category of mixed disorders should only be used when there is such an admixture that this cannot be done.

313.9   *Unspecified*

314   Hyperkinetic syndrome of childhood

Disorders in which the essential features are short attention-span and distractibility. In early childhood the most striking symptom is disinhibited, poorly organized and poorly regulated extreme overactivity but in adolescence this may be replaced by under-activity. Impulsiveness, marked mood fluctuations and aggression are also common symptoms. Delays in the development of specific skills are often present and disturbed, poor relationships are common. If the hyperkinesis is symptomatic of an underlying disorder, code the underlying disorder instead.

314.0   *Simple disturbance of activity and attention*

Cases in which short attention span, distractibility, and overactivity are the main manifestations without significant disturbance of conduct or delay in specific skills.

Overactivity NOS

314.1   *Hyperkinesis with developmental delay*

Cases in which the hyperkinetic syndrome is associated with speech delay, clumsiness, reading difficulties or other delays in specific skills.

Developmental disorder of hyperkinesis

Use additional code to identify any associated neurological disorder

314.2   *Hyperkinetic conduct disorder*

Cases in which the hyperkinetic syndrome is associated with marked conduct distur-bance but not developmental delay.

Hyperkinetic conduct disorder

Excludes: hyperkinesis with significant delays in specific skills (314.1)

314.8   *Other*

314.9   *Unspecified*

Hyperkinetic reaction of childhood   Hyperkinetic syndrome NOS
    or adolescence NOS

315   Specific delays in development

A group of disorders in which a specific delay in development is the main feature. In each case development is related to biological maturation but it is also influenced by nonbiological factors and the coding carries no aetiological implications.

Excludes: when due to a neurological disorder (320-389)

315.0   *Specific reading retardation*

Disorders in which the main feature is a serious impairment in the development of reading or spelling skills which is not explicable in terms of general intellectual retar-dation or of inadequate schooling. Speech or language difficulties, impaired right-left differentiation, perceptuo-motor problems, and coding difficulties are frequently asso-ciated. Similar problems are often present in other members of the family. Adverse psychosocial factors may be present.

Developmental dyslexia   Specific spelling difficulty

315.1   *Specific arithmetical retardation*

Disorders in which the main feature is a serious impairment in the development of arithmetical skills which is not explicable in terms of general intellectual retardation or of inadequate schooling.

Dyscalculia

315.2   *Other specific learning difficulties*

Disorders in which the main feature is a serious impairment in the development of other learning skills which are not explicable in terms of general intellectual retardation or of inadequate schooling.

Excludes: specific arithmetical retardation (315.1)
                   specific reading retardation (315.0)

315.3   *Developmental speech or language disorder*

Disorders in which the main feature is a serious impairment in the development of speech or language [syntax or semantics] which is not explicable in terms of general intellectual retardation. Most commonly there is a delay in the development of normal word-sound production resulting in defects of articulation. Omissions or substitutions of consonants are most frequent. There may also be a delay in the production of spoken language. Rarely, there is also a developmental delay in the comprehension of sounds. Includes cases in which delay is largely due to environmental privation.

Developmental aphasia   Dyslalia

Excludes: acquired aphasia (784.3)
                   elective mutism (309.8, 313.0 or 313.2)
                   lisping and lalling (307.9)
                   stammering and stuttering (307.0)

315.4   *Specific motor retardation*

Disorders in which the main feature is a serious impairment in the development of motor coordination which is not explicable in terms of general intellectual retardation. The clumsiness is commonly associated with perceptual difficulties.

Clumsiness syndrome   Dyspraxia syndrome

315.5   *Mixed development disorder*

A delay in the development of one specific skill [e.g., reading, arithmetic, speech or coordination] is frequently associated with lesser delays in other skills. When this occurs the coding should be made according to the skill most seriously impaired. The mixed category should be used only where the mixture of delayed skills is such that no one skill is preponderantly affected.

315.8   *Other*

315.9   *Unspecified*

Developmental disorder NOS

316   Psychic factors associated with diseases classified elsewhere

Mental disturbances or psychic factors of any type thought to have played a major part in the aetiology of physical conditions, usually involving tissue damage, classified elsewhere. The mental disturbance is usually mild and nonspecific and psychic factors [worry, fear, conflict, etc.] may be present without any overt psychiatric disorder. Use an additional code to identify the physical condition. In the rare instance that an overt psychiatric disorder is thought to have caused a physical condition, use a second additional code to record the psychiatric diagnosis.

Examples of the use of this category are:
  psychogenic:
      asthma 316 and 493.9
      dermatitis 316 and 692.–
      eczema 316 and 691.– or 692.–
      gastric ulcer 316 and 531.–
      mucous colitis 316 and 564.1
      ulcerative colitis 316 and 556
      urticaria 316 and 708.–
  psychosocial dwarfism 316 and 259.4

Excludes: physical symptoms and physiological malfunctions, not involving tissue damage, of mental origin (306.–)

MENTAL RETARDATION (317-319)

A condition of arrested or incomplete development of mind which is especially characterized by subnormality of intelligence. The coding should be made on the individual's *current* level of functioning *without regard to its nature* or causation—such as psychosis, cultural deprivation, Down's syndrome etc.. Where there is a specific cognitive handicap—such as in speech—the four-digit coding should be based on assessments of cognition *outside the area of specific handicap*. The assessment of intellectual level should be based on whatever information is available, including clinical evidence, adaptive behaviour and psychometric findings. The IQ levels given are based on a test with a mean of 100 and a standard deviation of 15—such as the Wechsler scales. They are provided only as a guide and should not be applied rigidly. Mental retardation often involves psychiatric disturbances and may often develop as a result of some physical disease or injury. In these cases, an additional code or codes should be used to identify any associated condition, psychiatric or physical. The Impairment and Handicap codes should also be consulted.

317   Mild mental retardation

Feeble-minded   Moron
High-grade defect   IQ 50-70
Mild mental subnormality

318   Other specified mental retardation

318.0 *Moderate mental retardation*

Imbecile   Moderate mental subnormality
IQ 35-49

318.1   *Severe mental retardation*

IQ 20-34   Severe mental subnormality

318.2   *Profound mental retardation*

Idiocy   Profound mental subnormality
IQ under 20

319   Unspecified mental retardation

Mental deficiency NOS   Mental subnormality NOS

Quick reference lists

QUICK REFERENCE LIST No. 1: ICD-9 CATEGORIES IN WHICH DEPRESSION IS A MAJOR OR SIGNIFICANT FEATURE

(10 3-digit categories: 19 4-digit categories)

QUICK REFERENCE LIST NO. 2:
NEW CATEGORIES SPECIFICALLY FOR DISORDERS OF CHILDHOOD AND ADOLESCENCE

The following new categories are provided in the ICD-9 specifically for disorders of childhood and adolescence. Other categories that are often, but not exclusively, applicable to children and adolescents can be found in: 307 "Special symptoms and syndromes not elsewhere classified"; in 309 "Adjustment reaction"; in 312 "Disturbance of conduct not elsewhere classified" (includes delinquency); and in categories 317–319, dealing with mental retardation.

QUICK REFERENCE LIST NO. 3:
ICD-8 AND ICD-9 EQUIVALENCES AND OMISSIONS

Equivalences between certain ICD-8 and ICD-9 3-digit categories

ICD-8	ICD-9
290 Senile and presenile dementia	290 Senile and presenile organic psychotic conditions
292 Psychosis associated with intracranial infection	
293 Psychosis associated with other cerebral condition	293 Transient organic psychotic conditions [*plus* additional code from elsewhere in ICD-9 for associated physical conditions]
294 Psychosis associated with other physical condition	294 Other organic psychotic conditions (chronic)
305 Physical disorders of presumably psychogenic origin	316 Psychic factors associated with diseases classified elsewhere [*plus* additional code]
307 Transient situational disturbances [no subdivisions]	308 Acute reaction to stress [with subdivisions]
	309 Adjustment reaction [with subdivisions]
308 Behaviour disorders of childhood [with suggested subdivisions for informal trial]	313 Disturbance of emotions specific to childhood and adolescence
	314 Hyperkinetic syndrome of childhood
	315 Specific delays in development [and parts of:]
	309 Ajustment reaction
	312 Disturbance of conduct not elsewhere classified
310 Borderline	317 Mild
311 Mild	318 Other specified	Mental retardation
312 Moderate Mental retardation	319 Unspecified
313 Severe	[*plus* use of additional code to specify associated physical conditions]
314 Profound	
315 Unspecified	

Some 3-digit categories in ICD-9 that were not in ICD-8

305   Nondependent abuse of drugs
308   Acute reaction to stress
309   Adjustment reaction
311   Depressive disorder, not elsewhere classified
312   Disturbance of conduct not elsewhere classified
316   Psychic factors associated with diseases classified elsewhere

The purposes and arrangement of the ICD-9 as a whole

Physicians, administrators and clerical workers who are responsible for establishing, recording or coding the diagnoses of psychiatric patients in terms of the chapter on mental disorders of the ICD-9 will often need to record the presence of additional physical conditions (such as infections, intoxications, or metabolic disorders) or external factors (such as trauma, poisonings, or acts of violence) covered by other chapters of the ICD; these are listed in Annex 3. The value of using the ICD to code multiple conditions presented by a patient is being increasingly recognized, and to encourage this practice there follows a brief introduction and guide to the ICD-9 as a whole. Those interested in further information should refer to the Introductions to Volumes 1 and 2 of the full ICD-9.[1]

Purposes and uses of the ICD

The ICD is a statistical classification of diseases; complications of pregnancy, childbirth, and the puerperium; congenital abnormalities; causes of perinatal morbidity and mortality; accidents, poisonings, and violence; and symptoms, signs, and ill-defined conditions. The principal use of the ICD is in the classification of morbidity and mortality information for statistical purposes. It has also been adapted for use as a nomenclature of diseases and in indexing medical records. The basic purpose of such indexing is to facilitate retrieval of medical records for a variety of purposes (for example, for studies of management of patients with specific conditions).

Organizational arrangement of the ICD-9

As stated in the Preface to the present volume, the ICD is a statistical classification of diseases and not a nomenclature of diseases. A nomenclature of diseases is a list or catalogue of approved terms for describing and recording clinical and pathological observations. To serve its full function it must be sufficiently extensive so that any pathological condition can be accurately recorded. As medical science advances a

---

[1] WORLD HEALTH ORGANIZATION. *Manual of the International Statistical Classification of Diseases, Injuries, and Causes of Death,* 1975 (Ninth) Revision, Geneva, Volumes 1 and 2, 1977 and 1978.

nomenclature must expand to include new terms necessary to record new observations. In contrast a statistical classification must be confined to a limited number of categories that encompass the entire range of disease and morbid conditions.

The ICD is organized in 17 major chapters (see Annex 2). Each of these is subdivided into a defined set of categories, identified by 3 digits, ranging from 000 to 999. Each such category is further divided into additional subcategories by a fourth digit (.0 to .9) so as to provide greater detail. The structure of the classification is eclectic in that the axes of classification are not consistent within each of the 17 major chapters. The primary axis is topographical in some of these categories (e.g., diseases of the respiratory system); less frequently it is etiological (e.g., infectious diseases) or situational (e.g., complications of pregnancy). In other sections, still other primary axes are used, reflecting the fact that the ICD is a compromise that provides a pragmatic classification that can be used for a variety of purposes. [1, 2]

There are also two supplementary chapters, one for classification of external causes of injury and poisoning (the E code) and the second for classification of factors influencing health status and contact with health services (the V code). Both of these classifications contain rubrics with items of relevance to agencies and facilities that provide psychiatric and related mental health services.

Revisions of the ICD

The revision of the ICD is a continuous process. As soon as one revision is completed, work starts on the next. In some instances, as with the mental disorders, work on the next revision starts well before work on the current revision is completed. Each revision requires an extensive set of activities; these include development of revision proposals by national agencies that compile health and vital statistics, bipartite or multipartite meetings of interested countries to develop joint proposals, coordination of programmes of the health agencies in different regions with the programmes of the WHO Centres for Classification of Diseases, convening expert committees to deal with various technical matters related to specific classification problems, and carrying out various types of special studies.

---

[1] SARTORIUS, N. Modifications and new approaches to taxonomy in long-term care: advantages and limitations of the ICD. *Medical care*, **14**: Suppl., pp. 109–115 (1976).

[2] KRAMER, M. The historical background of ICD-8. In: Committee on Nomenclature and Statistics. *Diagnostic and statistical manual of mental disorders (DSM-II)*, Washington, DC, American Psychiatric Association, 2nd ed., 1968, pp. xi–xv.

Of particular importance for the mental health field was Stengel's study[1] of the state of psychiatric classification throughout the world. He concluded that ICD-6 had failed to find general acceptance as far as psychiatry was concerned and that major improvements were necessary. Stengel's recommendations for action to remedy the situation were strongly supported by the WHO Scientific Group on Mental Health Research, which in 1964 recommended that WHO develop a classification of mental disorders internationally applicable and acceptable. The World Health Organization subsequently developed a programme to implement this recommendation (see Preface).[2]

The Alphabetical Index to ICD-9

Volume 2 of the ICD contains the Alphabetical Index to the tabular list of Volume 1 and assists the coder in determining the assignment of a given diagnosis to the appropriate category. For example, rubella occurring as a manifest disease in a person would be coded as 056 (Chapter I, Infections and Parasitic Diseases). Maternal rubella affecting a fetus (e.g. causing later mental retardation in a child) would be coded as 771.0 (Chapter XV, Certain Conditions originating in the Perinatal Period). Pneumococcal pneumonia would be coded as 481 (Chapter VIII, Diseases of the Respiratory System), while tuberculous pneumonia would be coded as 011.6 (Chapter I, Infections and Parasitic Diseases). Cerebral atherosclerosis would be coded as 437.0 (Chapter VII, Diseases of the Circulatory System), epilepsy as 345, and multiple sclerosis as 340 (both in Chapter VI, Diseases of the Nervous System and Sense Organs). Because of its exhaustive nature, the Index inevitably includes many imprecise and undesirable terms that are still occasionally encountered on medical records and for which coders need an indication of their assignment in the classification, if only to a rubric for residual or ill-defined conditions. The presence of a term in Volume 2 of the ICD should therefore not be taken as sanction for its use in good medical terminology.

---

[1] STENGEL, E. Classification of mental disorders. *Bulletin of the World Health Organization,* **21**: 601–663 (1959).

[2] KRAMER, M. ET AL. The ICD-9 classification of mental disorders: a review of its development and contents. *Acta psychiatrica scandinavica* (in press).

Summary listing of the chapters and major categories of the ICD-9

I. INFECTIOUS AND PARASITIC DISEASES [139 categories]

Intestinal infectious diseases (001–009)
Tuberculosis (010–018)
Zoonotic bacterial diseases (020–027)
Other bacterial diseases (030–041)
Poliomyelitis and other non-arthropod-borne viral diseases of central nervous system (045–049)
Viral diseases accompanied by exanthem (050–057)
Arthropod-borne viral diseases (060–066)
Other diseases due to viruses and Chlamydiae (070–079)
Rickettsioses and other arthropod-borne diseases (080–088)
Syphilis and other venereal diseases (090–099)
Other spirochaetal diseases (100–104)
Mycoses (110–118)
Helminthiases (120–129)
Other infectious and parasitic diseases (130–136)
Late effects of infectious and parasitic diseases (137–139)

II. NEOPLASMS [100 categories]

Malignant neoplasm of lip, oral cavity and pharynx (140–149)
Malignant neoplasm of digestive organs and peritoneum (150–159)
Malignant neoplasm of respiratory and intrathoracic organs (160–165)
Malignant neoplasm of bone, connective tissue, skin and breast (170–175)
Malignant neoplasm of genitourinary organs (179–189)
Malignant neoplasm of other and unspecified sites (190–199)
Malignant neoplasm of lymphatic and haematopoietic tissue (200–208)
Benign neoplasms (210–229)
Carcinoma in situ (230–234)
Neoplasms of uncertain behaviour (235–238)
Neoplasms of unspecified nature (239)

III. ENDOCRINE, NUTRITIONAL AND METABOLIC DISEASES AND IMMUNITY DISORDERS [40 categories]

Disorders of thyroid gland (240–246)
Diseases of other endocrine glands (250–259)
Nutritional deficiencies (260–269)
Other metabolic disorders and immunity disorders (270–279)

IV. DISEASES OF BLOOD AND BLOOD-FORMING ORGANS (280–289)
[10 categories]

V. MENTAL DISORDERS
[30 categories]

Organic psychotic conditions (290–294)
Other psychoses (295–299)
Neurotic disorders, personality disorders and other nonpsychotic mental disorders (300–316)
Mental retardation (317–319)

VI. DISEASES OF THE NERVOUS SYSTEM AND SENSE ORGANS
[70 categories]

Inflammatory diseases of the central nervous system (320–326)
Hereditary and degenerative diseases of the central nervous system (330–337)
Other disorders of the central nervous system (340–349)
Disorders of the peripheral nervous system (350–359)
Disorders of the eye and adnexa (360–379)
Diseases of the ear and mastoid process (380–389)

VII. DISEASES OF THE CIRCULATORY SYSTEM
[70 categories]

Acute rheumatic fever (390–392)
Chronic rheumatic heart disease (393–398)
Hypertensive disease (401–405)
Ischaemic heart disease (410–414)
Diseases of pulmonary circulation (415–417)
Other forms of heart disease (420–429)
Cerebrovascular disease (430–438)
Diseases of arteries, arterioles and capillaries (440–448)
Diseases of veins and lymphatics, and other diseases of circulatory system (451–459)

VIII. DISEASES OF THE RESPIRATORY SYSTEM
[60 categories]

Acute respiratory infections (460–466)
Other diseases of upper respiratory tract (470–478)
Pneumonia and influenza (480–487)
Chronic obstructive pulmonary disease and allied conditions (490–496)
Pneumoconioses and other lung diseases due to external agents (500–508)
Other diseases of respiratory system (510–519)

IX. DISEASES OF THE DIGESTIVE SYSTEM   [60 categories]

Diseases of oral cavity, salivary glands and jaws (520–529)
Diseases of oesophagus, stomach and duodenum (530–537)
Appendicitis (540–543)
Hernia of abdominal cavity (550–553)
Noninfective enteritis and colitis (555–558)
Other diseases of intestines and peritoneum (560–569)
Other diseases of digestive system (570–579)

X. DISEASES OF THE GENITOURINARY SYSTEM   [50 categories]

Nephritis, nephrotic syndrome and nephrosis (580–589)
Other diseases of urinary system (590–599)
Diseases of male genital organs (600–608)
Disorders of breast (610–611)
Inflammatory disease of female pelvic organs (614–616)
Other disorders of female genital tract (617–629)

XI. COMPLICATIONS OF PREGNANCY, CHILDBIRTH AND THE
PUERPERIUM   [50 categories]

Pregnancy with abortive outcome (630–639)
Complications mainly related to pregnancy (640–648)
Normal delivery, and other indications for care in pregnancy, labour and delivery
    (650–659)
Complications occurring mainly in the course of labour and delivery
    (660–669)
Complications of the puerperium (670–676)

XII. DISEASES OF THE SKIN
AND SUBCUTANEOUS TISSUE   [30 categories]

Infections of skin and subcutaneous tissue (680–686)
Other inflammatory conditions of skin and subcutaneous tissue (690–698)
Other diseases of skin and subcutaneous tissue (700–709)

XIII. DISEASES OF THE MUSCULOSKELETAL SYSTEM AND
CONNECTIVE TISSUE   [30 categories]

Arthropathies and related disorders (710–719)
Dorsopathies (720–724)
Rheumatism, excluding the back (725–729)
Osteopathies, chondropathies and acquired musculoskeletal deformities
    (730–739)

XIV. CONGENITAL ANOMALIES (740–759)   [20 categories]

XV. CERTAIN CONDITIONS ORIGINATING IN THE PERINATAL PERIOD (760–779)   [20 categories]

XVI. SYMPTOMS, SIGNS AND ILL-DEFINED CONDITIONS   [20 categories]

Symptoms (780–789)
Nonspecific abnormal findings (790–796)
Ill-defined and unknown causes of morbidity and mortality (797–799)

XVII. INJURY AND POISONING   [200 categories]

Fracture of skull (800–804)
Fracture of spine and trunk (805–809)
Fracture of upper limb (810–819)
Fracture of lower limb (820–829)
Dislocation (830–839)
Sprains and strains of joints and adjacent muscles (840–848)
Intracranial injury, excluding those with skull fracture (850–854)
Internal injury of chest, abdomen and pelvis (860–869)
Open wound of head, neck and trunk (870–879)
Open wound of upper limb (880–887)
Open wound of lower limb (890–897)
Injury to blood vessels (900–904)
Late effects of injuries, poisonings, toxic effects and other external causes (905–909)
Superficial injury (910–919)
Contusion with intact skin surface (920–924)
Crushing injury (925–929)
Effects of foreign body entering through orifice (930–939)
Burns (940–949)
Injury to nerves and spinal cord (950–957)
Certain traumatic complications and unspecified injuries (958–959)
Poisoning by drugs, medicaments and biological substances (960–979)
Toxic effects of substances chiefly nonmedicinal as to source (980–989)
Other and unspecified effects of external causes (990–995)
Complications of surgical and medical care not elsewhere classified (996–999)

SUPPLEMENTARY CLASSIFICATION OF EXTERNAL CAUSES OF INJURY AND POISONING   [1000 categories]

Railway accidents (E800–E807)
Motor vehicle traffic accidents (E810–E819)
Motor vehicle nontraffic accidents (E820–E825)

Other road vehicle accidents (E826–E829)
Water transport accidents (E830–E838)
Air and space transport accidents (E840–E845)
Vehicle accidents not elsewhere classifiable (E846–E848)
Accidental poisoning by drugs, medicaments and biologicals (E850–E858)
Accidental poisoning by other solid and liquid substances, gases and vapours
    (E860–E869)
Misadventures to patients during surgical and medical care (E870–E876)
Surgical and medical procedures as the cause of abnormal reaction of patient or
    later complication, without mention of misadventure at the time of
    procedure (E878–E879)
Accidental falls (E880–E888)
Accidents caused by fire and flames (E890–E899)
Accidents due to natural and environmental factors (E900–E909)
Accidents caused by submersion, suffocation and foreign bodies (E910–E915)
Other accidents (E916–E928)
Late effects of accidental injury (E929)
Drugs, medicaments and biological substances causing adverse effects in thera-
    peutic use (E930–E949)
Suicide and selfinflicted injury (E950–E959)
Homicide and injury purposely inflicted by other persons (E960–E969)
Legal intervention (E970–E978)
Injury undetermined whether accidentally or purposely inflicted (E980–E989)
Injury resulting from operations of war (E990–E999)

SUPPLEMENTARY CLASSIFICATION OF FACTORS INFLUENCING HEALTH STATUS AND CONTACT WITH HEALTH SERVICES

[82 categories]

Persons with potential health hazards related to communicable diseases
    (V01–V07)
Persons with potential health hazards related to personal and family history
    (V10–V19)
Persons encountering health services in circumstances related to reproduction
    and development (V20–V28)
Healthy liveborn infants according to type of birth (V30–V39)
Persons with a condition influencing their health status (V40–V49)
Persons encountering health services for specific procedures and aftercare
    (V50–V59)
Persons encountering health services in other circumstances (V60–V68) ·
Persons without reported diagnosis encountered during examination and investi-
    gation of individuals and populations (V70–V82)

Conditions in the ICD-9 outside Chapter V that can give rise to psychiatric disorders or lead to contact with the psychiatric services

For the convenience of diagnosticians and coders, who may not always have ready access to the complete ICD volumes, those conditions outside Chapter V most commonly giving rise to contacts with psychiatric services are listed below with their codes. This list is not comprehensive but it will be found to cover the great majority of cases encountered in ordinary psychiatric practice.

The Ninth Revision of the ICD uses two codes for certain diagnostic descriptions which contain information about a localized manifestation or complication and about a more generalized underlying disease process. The code for the latter is marked with a dagger (†), and for the former with an asterisk (*). Thus tuberculous meningitis has its dagger code in the chapter for infectious and parasitic diseases and its asterisk code in the nervous systems chapter.

I. INFECTIOUS AND PARASITIC DISEASES [1]

006 Amoebiasis

006.5 *Amoebic brain abscess*

013 Tuberculosis of meninges and central nervous system

013.0 † *Tuberculous meningitis (320.4*)*
013.1 † *Tuberculoma of meninges (349.2*)*
013.8 Tuberculoma † ⎫
        Tuberculosis † ⎭ of brain (348.8*)
        Tuberculous:
          abscess of brain † (324.0*)

027 Other zoonotic bacterial diseases

027.0 Meningitis † (320.7*) ⎫
       Meningoencephalitis † (320.7*) ⎭ by Listeria monocytogenes

---

[1] Headings of 4-digit categories in ICD-9 are italicized in this list; inclusion terms are not.

036   Meningococcal infection

036.0 †   *Meningococcal meningitis (320.5*)*
036.1 †   *Meningococcal encephalitis (323.4*)*

046   Slow virus infection of central nervous system

046.0 †   *Kuru (323.0*)*
046.1 †   *Jakob-Creutzfeldt disease (331.5*)*
046.3 †   *Progressive multifocal leucoencephalopathy (331.6*)*

047   Meningitis due to enterovirus

047.0 †   *Coxsackie virus (321.1*)*
047.1 †   *ECHO virus (321.2*)*
047.8 †   *Other (321.7*)*
047.9 †   Viral meningitis NOS (321.7*)

**049   Other non-arthropod-borne viral diseases of central nervous
               system**

049.0 †   *Lymphocytic choriomeningitis (321.6*)*
049.1 †   *Meningitis due to adenovirus (321.7*)*
049.8   Encephalitis: acute
049.9   Viral encephalitis NOS † (323.4*)

054   Herpes simplex

054.3 †   *Herpetic meningoencephalitis (323.4*)*
054.7   Meningitis due to herpes simplex † (321.4*)

090   Congenital syphilis

090.4   *Juvenile neurosyphilis*

094   Neurosyphilis

094.0   *Tabes dorsalis*
094.1   *General paresis*
094.2 †   *Syphilitic meningitis (320.7*)*
094.8   Syphilitic: encephalitis † (323.4*)

130   Toxoplasmosis

          Meningoencephalitis † (323.4*) due to acquired
          toxoplasmosis

137   Late effects of tuberculosis

137.1   *Late effects of central nervous system tuberculosis*

139   **Late effects of other infectious and parasitic diseases**

139.0   *Late effects of viral encephalitis*

II.   NEOPLASMS

191   **Malignant neoplasm of brain**

192   **Malignant neoplasm of other and unspecified parts of nervous system**

192.1   *Cerebral meninges*

198   **Secondary malignant neoplasm of other specified sites**

198.3   *Brain and spinal cord*
198.4   Meninges (cerebral)

225   **Benign neoplasm of brain and other parts of nervous system**

225.0   *Brain*
225.2   *Cerebral meninges*

237   **Neoplasm of uncertain behaviour of endocrine glands and nervous system**

237.5   *Brain and spinal cord*
237.6   *Meninges*

239   **Neoplasms of unspecified nature**

239.6   Brain
          Excludes cerebral meninges (239.7)
239.7   *Endocrine glands, and other parts of nervous system*

III.   ENDOCRINE, NUTRITIONAL AND METABOLIC DISEASES AND IMMUNITY DISORDERS

242   **Thyrotoxicosis with or without goitre**

242.0   *Toxic diffuse goitre*
242.9   Hyperthyroidism NOS
243   *Congenital hypothyroidism*
          Congenital thyroid insufficiency
          Cretinism
          Use additional code if desired, to identify associated mental retardation

244   **Acquired hypothyroidism**

244.9   Myxoedema, primary or NOS

251   **Disorders of pancreatic internal secretion other than diabetes mellitus**

251.2   *Hypoglycaemia, unspecified*

253   **Diseases of pituitary gland and its hypothalamic control**

253.0   *Acromegaly and gigantism*
253.3   *Pituitary dwarfism*
253.8   Fröhlich's syndrome

259   **Other endocrine disorders**

259.4   *Dwarfism, not elsewhere classified*
259.9   Infantilism NOS

270   **Disorders of amino-acid transport and metabolism**

270.1   *Phenylketonuria*
270.3   Maple-syrup-urine disease

271   **Disorders of carbohydrate transport and metabolism**

271.1   *Galactosaemia*

275   **Disorders of mineral metabolism**

275.1   Hepatolenticular degeneration

277   **Other and unspecified disorders of metabolism**

277.1   *Disorders of porphyrin metabolism*
          Porphyria
277.5   *Mucopolysaccharidosis*
          Gargoylism

VI. DISEASES OF THE NERVOUS SYSTEM AND SENSE ORGANS

320   **Bacterial meningitis**

320.4*   *Tuberculous meningitis* (013.0 †)
320.5   *Meningococcal meningitis* (036.0 †)

323   Encephalitis, myelitis and encephalomyelitis

323.0*   *Kuru* (046.0 †)
323.7*   *Toxic encephalitis*
           Lead encephalitis (984.– †)

330   Cerebral degenerations usually manifest in childhood

330.0   *Leucodystrophy*
330.1   *Cerebral lipidoses*
           Amaurotic (family) idiocy
           Tay-Sachs disease

331   Other cerebral degenerations

331.0   *Alzheimer's disease*
331.1   *Pick's disease*
331.2   *Senile degeneration of the brain*
           Excludes: senility NOS (797)
331.5*   *Jakob-Creutzfeldt disease* (046.1 †)
331.6*   *Progressive multifocal leucoencephalopathy* (046.3 †)
331.7*   *Cerebral degeneration in other disease classified elsewhere*
           in alcoholism (303 †)
           in beriberi (265.0 †)
           in congenital hydrocephalus (741.0, 742.3 †)
           in myxoedema (244.– †)

333   Other extrapyramidal disease and abnormal movement disorders

333.4   *Huntington's chorea*

334   Spinocerebellar disease

334.0   *Friedreich's ataxia*

341   Other demyelinating diseases of central nervous system

341.1   *Schilder's disease*

345   Epilepsy

345.0   *Generalized nonconvulsive epilepsy*
345.1   *Generalized convulsive epilepsy*
345.2   *Petit mal status*
345.3   *Grand mal status*
345.4   *Partial epilepsy, with impairment of consciousness*

345.5   *Partial epilepsy, without mention of impairment of conscious-*
         ness
345.6   *Infantile spasms*
345.7   *Epilepsia partialis continua*
345.8   *Other*
345.9   *Unspecified*
         Epileptic convulsions, fits or seizures NOS

346   Migraine

347   Cataplexy and narcolepsy

348   Other conditions of brain

348.1   *Anoxic brain damage*
348.3   *Encephalopathy, unspecified*
348.8   *Other*
         Cerebral:
            calcification
            fungus
         Tuberculoma ⎫ of brain (active disease)* (013.8 †)
         Tuberculosis ⎭

IX.   DISEASES OF THE DIGESTIVE SYSTEM

571   Chronic liver disease and cirrhosis

571.0   *Alcoholic fatty liver*
571.1   *Acute alcoholic hepatitis*
571.2   *Alcoholic cirrhosis of liver*
         Laënnec's cirrhosis
571.3   *Alcoholic liver damage, unspecified*

X.   DISEASES OF THE GENITOURINARY SYSTEM

**625   Pain and other symptoms associated with female genital
          organs**

625.4   *Premenstrual tension syndromes*
625.6   *Stress incontinence, female*

627   Menopausal and postmenopausal disorders

         Symptoms such as flushing, sleeplessness, headache, lack of
         concentration, associated with the menopause

XI. COMPLICATIONS OF PREGNANCY, CHILDBIRTH AND THE PUERPERIUM

648 **Other current conditions in the mother classifiable elsewhere, but complicating pregnancy, childbirth and the puerperium**

648.3 *Drug dependence*
Conditions in 304.–

648.4 *Mental disorders*
Conditions in 290–303, 305–316, 317–319

XIV. CONGENITAL ANOMALIES

740 **Anencephalus and similar anomalies**

740.0 *Anencephalus*

741 **Spina bifida**

741.0 *With hydrocephalus*

742 **Other congenital abnormalities of nervous system**

742.1 *Microcephalus*

742.3 *Congenital hydrocephalus*
Excludes hydrocephalus:
acquired (331.4)
due to congenital toxoplasmosis (771.2 †, 331.4*)

742.4 *Other specified anomalies of brain*
Congenital cerebral cyst
Megalencephaly
Multiple anomalies of brain NOS

742.9 *Unspecified anomalies of brain, spinal cord and nervous system*
Anomaly
Congenital disease or lesion } of brain
Deformity

756 **Certain congenital musculoskeletal deformities**

756.0 *Anomalies of skull and face bones*
Craniosynostosis
Hypertelorism

758   **Chromosomal abnormalities**

758.0   *Down's syndrome*
           Trisomy:
               21 or 22
               G
758.1   *Patau's syndrome*
           Trisomy:
               13
               D₁
758.2   *Edwards's syndrome*
           Trisomy:
               18
               E₃
758.6   *Gonadal dysgenesis*
           Turner's syndrome
           XO syndrome
               Excludes pure gonadal dysgenesis (752.7)
758.7   *Klinefelter's syndrome*
           XXY syndrome
758.8   *Other conditions due to sex chromosome anomalies*

759   **Other and unspecified congenital anomalies**

759.5   *Tuberous sclerosis*
           Bourneville's disease
           Epiloia
759.6   *Other hamartoses, not elsewhere classified*
           Sturge-Weber (-Dimitri) syndrome

XVI.   SYMPTOMS, SIGNS AND ILL-DEFINED CONDITIONS

780   **General symptoms**

780.0   *Coma and stupor*
780.1   *Hallucinations*
               Excludes: visual hallucinations (368.1)
                             when part of a pattern of mental disorder
780.3   *Convulsions*
               Excludes: convulsions in newborn (779.0)
                             epileptic convulsions (345.–)
780.9   *Other*
           Amnesia (retrograde)
               Excludes: memory disturbance when part of a pattern of
               mental disorder

783 **Symptoms concerning nutrition, metabolism and development**

783.0 *Anorexia*
Loss of appetite
Excludes: anorexia nervosa (307.1)
loss of appetite of nonorganic origin (307.5)

784 **Symptoms involving head and neck**

784.3 *Aphasia*
784.5 *Other speech disturbance*
Dysphasia
784.6 *Other symbolic dysfunction*
Agraphia
Dyslexia
Excludes: developmental learning retardations (315.–)

788 **Symptoms involving urinary system**

788.3 *Incontinence of urine*
Enuresis NOS
Excludes: when of nonorganic origin (307.6)
stress incontinence (female) (625.6)

799 **Other ill-defined and unknown causes of morbidity and mortality**

799.2 *Nervousness*

XVII. INJURY AND POISONING

850 **Concussion**

851 **Cerebral laceration and contusion**

852 **Subarachnoid, subdural and extradural haemorrhage, following injury**

853 **Other and unspecified intracranial haemorrhage following injury**

854 **Intracranial injury of other and unspecified nature**

960 **Poisoning by antibiotics**

961 **Poisoning by other anti-infectives**

962   Poisoning by hormones and synthetic substitutes

963   Poisoning by primarily systemic agents

964   Poisoning by agents primarily affecting blood constituents

965   Poisoning by analgesics, antipyretics and antirheumatics

966   Poisoning by anticonvulsants and anti-Parkinsonism drugs

967   Poisoning by sedatives and hypnotics

968   Poisoning by other central nervous system depressants

969   Poisoning by psychotropic drugs

970   Poisoning by central nervous system stimulants

971   Poisoning by drugs primarily affecting the autonomic nervous system

972   Poisoning by agents primarily affecting the cardiovascular system

973   Poisoning by agents primarily affecting the gastrointestinal system

974   Poisoning by water, mineral and uric acid metabolism drugs

975   Poisoning by agents primarily acting on the smooth and skeletal muscles and respiratory system

976   Poisoning by agents primarily affecting skin and mucous membrane, ophthalmological, otorhinolaryngological and dental drugs

977   Poisoning by other and unspecified drugs and medicaments

978   Poisoning by bacterial vaccines

979   Poisoning by other vaccines and biological substances

980   Toxic effect of alcohol

981   Toxic effect of petroleum products

982   Toxic effect of solvents other than petroleum-based

983   Toxic effect of corrosive aromatics, acids and caustic alkalis

984   Toxic effect of lead and its compounds (including fumes)

985   Toxic effect of other metals

986   Toxic effect of carbon monoxide

987   Toxic effect of other gases, fumes or vapours

988   Toxic effect of noxious substances eaten as food

989   Toxic effect of other substances, chiefly nonmedicinal as to
            source

994   Effects of other external causes

994.2   *Effects of hunger*
          Deprivation of food
          Starvation

995   Certain adverse effects not elsewhere classified

995.5   *Child maltreatment syndrome*
          Battered baby or child syndrome NOS
          Emotional and/or nutritional maltreatment of child

999   Complications of medical care, not elsewhere classified

999.6   *ABO incompatibility reaction*
999.7   *Rh incompatibility reaction*
999.8   *Other transfusion reaction*
999.9   Other or unspecified misadventure of medical care

SUPPLEMENTARY CLASSIFICATION
OF EXTERNAL CAUSES
OF INJURY AND POISONING

E904   **Hunger, thirst, exposure, neglect**

E904.0   *Abandonment or neglect of infants and helpless persons*

E950   **Suicide and selfinflicted poisoning by solid or liquid substances**

E950.0   *Analgesics, antipyretics and antirheumatics*
E950.1   *Barbiturates*
E950.2   *Other sedatives and hypnotics*
E950.3   *Tranquillizers and other psychotropic agents*
E950.4   *Other specified drugs and medicaments*
E950.5   *Unspecified drug or medicament*
E950.6   *Agricultural and horticultural chemical and pharmaceutical preparations other than plant foods and fertilizers*
E950.7   *Corrosive and caustic substances*
E950.8   *Arsenic and its compounds*
E950.9   *Other and unspecified solid and liquid substances*

E951   **Suicide and selfinflicted poisoning by gases in domestic use**

E952   **Suicide and selfinflicted poisoning by other gases and vapours**

E953   **Suicide and selfinflicted injury by hanging, strangulation and suffocation**

E954   **Suicide and selfinflicted injury by submersion [drowning]**

E955   **Suicide and selfinflicted injury by firearms and explosives**

E956   **Suicide and selfinflicted injury by cutting and piercing instruments**

E957   **Suicide and selfinflicted injury by jumping from high places**

E958   **Suicide and selfinflicted injury by other and unspecified means**

SUPPLEMENTARY CLASSIFICATION OF FACTORS INFLUENCING HEALTH STATUS AND CONTACT WITH HEALTH SERVICES

V11   **Personal history of mental disorder**

V15   **Other personal history presenting hazards to health**

V15.4   *Psychological trauma*

V17   **Family history of certain chronic disabling diseases**

V17.0   *Psychiatric condition*
V17.2   *Other neurological diseases*
            Epilepsy
            Huntington's chorea

V18   **Family history of certain other specific conditions**

V18.4   *Mental retardation*

V26   **Procreative management**

V26.3   *Genetic counselling*
V26.4   *General counselling and advice*

V40   **Mental and behavioural problems**

V40.0   *Problems with learning*
V40.1   *Problems with communication [including speech]*
V40.2   *Other mental problems*
V40.3   *Other behavioural problems*
V40.9   *Unspecified mental or behavioural problems*

V41   **Problems with special senses and other special functions**

V41.7   *Problems with sexual function*

V57   **Care involving use of rehabilitation procedures**

V57.0   *Breathing exercises*
V57.1   *Other physical therapy*
V57.2   *Occupational therapy and vocational rehabilitation*
V57.3   *Speech therapy*

V60   **Housing, household and economic circumstances**

V60.4   *No other household member able to render care*
V60.5   *Holiday relief care*

V61   **Other family circumstances**

V61.0   *Family disruption*
V61.1   *Marital problems*
             Excludes: problems related to:
                        psychosexual disorders (302.–)
                        sexual functions (V41.7)
V61.2   *Parent-child problems*
V61.4   *Health problems within family*
             Alcoholism in family

V62   **Other psychosocial circumstances**

V62.1   *Adverse effects of work environment*
V62.3   Educational handicap

V66   **Convalescence**

V66.3   *Following psychotherapy and other treatment for mental disorder*

V67   **Follow-up examination**

V67.3   *Following psychotherapy and other treatment for mental disorder*

V68   **Encounters for administrative purposes**

V68.2   *Requests for expert evidence*

V70   **General medical examination**

V70.1   *General psychiatric examination, requested by the authority*
V70.2   *General psychiatric examination, other and unspecified*

V77   **Special screening for endocrine, nutritional, metabolic and immunity disorders**

V77.3   *Phenylketonuria*

V79   **Special screening for mental disorders and developmental handicaps**

V79.0   *Depression*
V79.1   *Alcoholism*
V79.2   *Mental retardation*

V82   **Special screening for other conditions**

V82.4   *Postnatal screening for chromosomal abnormalities*

Index

Abandonment or neglect of infants and helpless persons, 80
Abnormal movement disorders, 73
Absinthe addiction, 43
Acromegaly and gigantism, 72
Acute
  confusional state, 25
    delirium, 25
    infective psychosis, 25
    organic reaction, 25
    post-traumatic organic psychosis, 25
    psycho-organic syndrome, 25
    psychosis associated with endocrine, metabolic or cerebrovascular disorder, 25
    senile dementia, 23
  drunkenness in alcoholism, 42
  paranoid reaction, 33
  reaction to stress, 48–49
    mixed, 48
    unspecified, 49
  schizophrenia (undifferentiated), 29
  schizophrenic
    attack, 28
    episode, 28
  situational disturbance, 48
Adaptation reaction NOS, 50
Adjustment reaction, 49–50
  NOS, 50
Adolescence
  disturbance of emotions, 53
  hyperkinetic reaction NOS, 54
  withdrawing reaction, 53
Aerophagy, 45
Affective
  and paranoid organic psychotic states, mixed, 26
  personality disorder, 38
  psychoses, 29–31
  psychosis and schizophrenia, mixed, 29
  psychosis NOS, 31
  type schizophreniform psychosis, 29
Aggressive
  personality, 39
  reaction, 39
Agoraphobia, 36
Agraphia, 77
Agricultural and horticultural chemicals, in suicide and selfinflicted poisoning, 80

Air hunger, 44
Alcohol
  excessive drinking NOS, 43
  dependence syndrome, 42
  intoxication, 43
  toxic effect, 78
  withdrawal syndrome, 24
Alcoholic
  brain syndrome, chronic, 24
  cirrhosis of liver, 74
  delirium, 23
  dementia NOS, 24
  fatty liver, 74
  hallucinosis, 24
  "hangover", 43
  hepatitis, acute, 74
  jealousy, 24
  liver damage, unspecified, 74
  mania NOS, 24
  paranoia, 24
  polyneuritic psychosis, 23
  psychosis NOS, 24
Alcoholism, 82
  acute drunkenness, 42
  cerebral degeneration, 73
  chronic, 42
    with psychosis, 24
  in family, 82
Alzheimer's disease, 22, 73
Amino-acid transport and metabolism, disorders, 72
Amnesia, retrograde, 76
Amoebiasis, 69
Amoebic brain abscess, 69
Amoral personality, 40
Amphetamines, 24–25
Analgesics, in suicide and selfinflicted poisoning, 80
Anankastic
  neurosis, 36
  personality disorder, 39
Anencephalus and similar anomalies, 75
Animal phobias, 36
Anorexia, 77
  nervosa, 46
Antisocial personality, 40
Antipyretics, in suicide and selfinflicted poisoning, 80